Causation in Population Health Informatics and Data Science

Olaf Dammann • Benjamin Smart

Causation in Population Health Informatics and Data Science

Springer

Olaf Dammann
Department of Public Health and
Community Medicine
Tufts University School of Medicine
Boston, MA
USA

Benjamin Smart
The African Centre for Epistemology
and Philosophy of Science
University of Johannesburg
Johannesburg
South Africa

ISBN 978-3-030-07174-5 ISBN 978-3-319-96307-5 (eBook)
https://doi.org/10.1007/978-3-319-96307-5

This Springer imprint is published by the registered company Springer Nature Switzerland AG
The registered company address is: Gewerbestrasse 11, 6330 Cham, Switzerland

Preface

Human civilization as we know it would look very different were it not for collective efforts to maintain and improve population health. Access to the means that support individual and community health is a human right. The continued improvement of global public health must be an administrative and political priority, at local, regional, and national levels. So many health administrators, scientists, field workers, students, project coordinators, nurses, and physicians work tirelessly toward that goal. Better population health means better lives.

Academic schools and departments of medicine and public health are charged with the generation of new knowledge to help with this endeavor. Because effective medical and public health practice needs a solid scientific foundation, we need to devise methods that ensure the generation of unbiased data, reliable information, solid evidence, and useful knowledge. Most of these methods are computer-based; informatics and data science thus play a crucial role in this research. Accordingly, considerable attention has been paid over the past decade to the development of public health informatics, with the second edition of a comprehensive textbook [1] and the creation of an academic journal, the *Online Journal of Public Health Informatics* (ojphi.org). Most recently, *Population Health Informatics* has been added to the mix [2]. The field covers a broad variety of informatics applications in population health research and practice. One crucial issue, however, is the lack of substantial effort to improve the *interpretation* of population health data and inference, i.e., the generation of new knowledge [3, p. 100–1]. The central issue here is the lack of methods for interpretation and inference that help turn data into information, information into evidence, and evidence into knowledge.

This is the void this book attempts to fill, by bringing in a third perspective that comes from the growing interest among philosophers in causal explanation and mechanisms in the health sciences. Imagine a Venn diagram with three circles: one is informatics and data science, the second is the health sciences, and the third is philosophy of science. The topic of this book is situated right in the middle of the multidisciplinary space defined by the diagram, where all three circles overlap and where, as of yet, not much has been published.

This book had a lengthy gestation and many have helped along the way. Olaf Dammann would like to thank Guanglan Zhang, Naftali Weinberger, Olaf Wolkenhauer, Alex Broadbent, Ted Poston, Paul Thagard, and all his students and colleagues at Tufts for many interesting and helpful discussions. First and foremost though, a big thanks to Christiane, Lina, and Laura for their love, patience, and support. Benjamin Smart would like to thank Veli Mitova and Michael Talibard for their comments on earlier versions of Chaps. 3 and 4, Em Watson for her love and support, and his coauthor for relentless patience. Both authors appreciate the continued guidance offered by our editor Grant Weston at Springer.

We hope to generate a fruitful debate that will develop some of the ideas discussed in this book. We have tried to offer food for thought in a palatable way, and all errors are ours. Our last chapter is a standing invitation to contact us to join the conversation. As the chef of a good restaurant would say, if you don't like our food, tell us; if you do, tell others.

References

1. Magnuson JA, Fu PC. Public health informatics and information systems, Health informatics series. New York: Springer; 2014.
2. Joshi A, Thorpe L, Waldron L. Population health informatics: driving evidence-based solutions into practice. Burlington, Massachusetts: Jones & Bartlett Learning; 2019.
3. Tulchinsky TH, Varavikova E. The new public health. 2nd ed. Amsterdam/Boston: Elsevier/Academic Press; 2009. xxiv, 672 p.

Boston, MA, USA — Olaf Dammann
Johannesburg, South Africa — Benjamin Smart

Contents

Chapter 1
Introduction

Abstract The goal of this book is to take a first step towards a framework for causal explanation in public/population health informatics and analytics. We first provide an introduction to the concepts of public health informatics (PHI) and population health informatics (PopHI). Next, we introduce the general approach we take – the etiological stance – and the idea that risk and causation are two ways of looking at etiology, the process of illness occurrence. We offer a brief description of how the discussion of causation and causal inference in epidemiology relates to concepts in philosophy of science and contrast deterministic folk psychology of causation with a pragmatic perspective built on probabilistic concepts of causation. Finally, we clarify the agenda of this book with a focus on what it is not about and give a road-map of the remaining chapters.

Keywords Public health · Population health · Informatics · Etiology · Causation

The Patient Protection and Affordable Care Act is a 906 page federal statute that was signed into law on March 23rd, 2010. It introduced broad and substantial changes to health care provision and insurance in the United States.[1] The law was expected to yield far ranging consequences for the public's health.

In 2011, the Institutes of Medicine's (IOM) Committee on Public Health Strategies to Improve Health was asked to respond to three charges. The first was to review population health strategies and metrics within the framework of health care system reform. The second was to assess the effect of health statutes and regulations on population health measures, and the third was to suggest recommendations for population health support funding in the context of health care reform. The committee summarized its responses to each of the charges in three reports entitled *For the Public's Health.* The first report was sub-titled *The Role of Measurement in Action and Accountability* and it "suggests measurement strategies that would heighten accountability and galvanize broader action by communities and other stakeholders" [4:xv].

---

[1] https://www.gpo.gov/fdsys/granule/PLAW-111publ148/PLAW-111publ148/content-detail.html; accessed 4/7/2017.

O. Dammann, B. Smart, *Causation in Population Health Informatics and Data Science*, https://doi.org/10.1007/978-3-319-96307-5_1

The key words in this quotation are *measurement* and *action*, and both concepts are of crucial importance for this book.

One theoretical issue emphasized in the IOM report is the difficulty associated with causal inference and explanation, e.g., the need to use "data to derive or develop myriad indicators of the various dimensions of population health – from distal outcomes to underlying and intermediate causal factors" [4:10]. In keeping with this notion, our main position outlined in this book is that extracting meaning from collected data, putting them in context, and finding out how they relate to one another, is frequently identical to giving a *causal explanation.* Our goal is to make a first step towards a framework for causal explanation in public/population health informatics.

1.1 Background

We think about health and illness for at least two reasons. First, humans are notoriously self-centred. We have a vested interested in our own wellbeing and in maximizing our likelihood of survival. Second, despite all egotism, humans are also social creatures. As a collective, we depend on one another. Therefore, we also have a vested interest in the wellbeing of others in our local and wider communities. Both interests motivate us to avoid being mere bystanders in a world of ever changing, and arguably worsening, health risks. To reach our goals of personal and collective wellbeing, we have to do something.

We have to think about ways how to manage such risks proactively. Because we do not want to accept illness, resulting from diseases, disorders, and accidents and their consequences as something given, inevitable, and unchangeable, we have agreed on effective ways to take action. Let's call this the *interventionist stance* of medicine and public health. Medicine is devoted to the reduction of suffering by treating illness pharmacologically, psychologically, or surgically, while public health efforts focus on interventions designed to reduce the effects of health hazards via prevention.[2]

All attempts to maintain and improve population health are, taken together, the backdrop for this book. This kind of work is performed at local, regional, national, and global levels. Public Health Informatics (PHI) plays an increasingly important role at all these levels.

One recent development we need to consider here is the expansion of scope that comes with moving from PHI to population health informatics (PopHI) [5]. In this proposed framework, PHI is the application of health information science and technology in the *total* population (excluding the health care system), while PopHI) refers to total and *specified* populations as well as healthcare system and provider organizations (Fig. 1.1). In this book, we take an inclusive perspective: our focus is on PHI; however, most concepts related to causal inference and explanation are transferrable to PopHI) without much need for adjustment.

[2] Both are at their best when considered health management in a non-commercial sense that should be available, affordable to all without considerations about revenues and losses for health care providers and insurances.

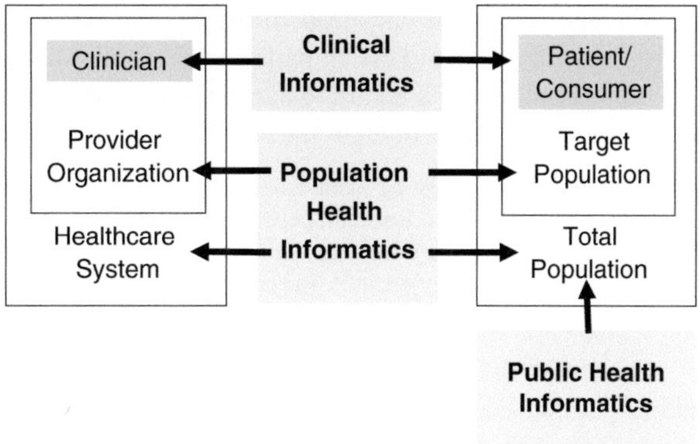

Fig. 1.1 The scope of clinical informatics, population health informatics, and public health informatics. (Modified from Kharrazi et al. [5])

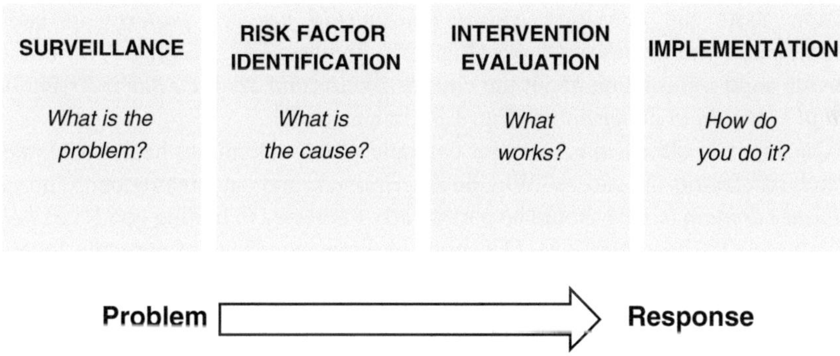

Fig. 1.2 The public health approach requires causal explanation at all levels, with a particular focus on risk factor identification. (Modified from https://www.cdc.gov/publichealth101/documents/introduction-to-public-health.pdf; slides in the public domain)

In this book, we ask, "What role does causal explanation play in Public/Population Health Informatics and Data Science"? Our goal is to shed light onto this one particular facet of population health management and research, causal explanation, that we think has so far been largely neglected, although risk factor identification is an integral part of the public health approach (Fig. 1.2). We frequently write from the medical perspective, and from the perspective of philosophy of medicine. This is mainly because the philosophy of medicine literature is considerably larger than the literature of philosophy of population health.

Health Informatics is concerned with the collection, storage, organization, distribution, and analysis of health data. One formal definition of *Public Health Informatics* is this:

Definition *Public Health Informatics* is the application of information science and technology to public health practice and research [6:240]

The scope of PHI includes "the conceptualization, design, development, deployment, refinement maintenance, and evaluation of communication surveillance, information systems, and learning systems relevant to public health" [1:4].

Situated before this backdrop, this book provides commentary on theoretical, causation-related issues in PHI. In part, it is a response to calls for more theory in public health informatics with regard to data analysis and interpretation. For example, Rolka and colleagues have written in the context of public health surveillance that

> integrating and analyzing data from new and multiple sources pose new challenges. A major reason is that time and experience are fundamental to learning about the data, the system, how to prepare the data for analysis, and to analyze the data and create reports, often on a rapid cyclic schedule. In certain instances, the required work has never been done before [7].

Most work in PHI makes use of methods and tools that provide valid information about population health, which – in turn – can be used as a basis for public health interventions that work. To achieve this goal, PHI needs to provide valid information about two dimensions of public health: First, PHI needs to deliver valid information about the purported *causal relationship between patterns of health determinants and health outcomes* (Fig. 1.3, dimension A). Second, PHI needs to provide solid information about the *causal relationship between our interventions and phenomena in dimension A* (Fig. 1.3, dimension B).

Questions in dimension A are, for example, What determines health outcomes? Which risk factors are causes? Why do determinants and outcomes occur? The *surveillance domain* of PHI should be particularly interested in finding good (i.e., *helpful*) answers to these questions. Questions in dimension B are of particular interest to those who work in the *evaluation domain* of PHI. In a sense, we want to know precisely what is going on in the population that leads to changes in its health (domain/dimension A) and what we can do about it (B)? Observable changes in the observable characteristics of causal processes in populations are all we have to answer those questions. We want to reinforce the beneficial processes in order to promote health, and interfere with detrimental ones to prevent their potential undesirable health consequences. Most importantly, we want these interventions to be effective. We want them to work.

Public Health Informatics provides tools and concepts that support this mission [1, 2]. The field is developing rapidly in parallel with other areas of biomedical informatics. All data-related aspects of public health administration and research in Departments of Public Health, academia, and the health care sector, are undergoing constant change, moving from data collection on paper to electronic records, from

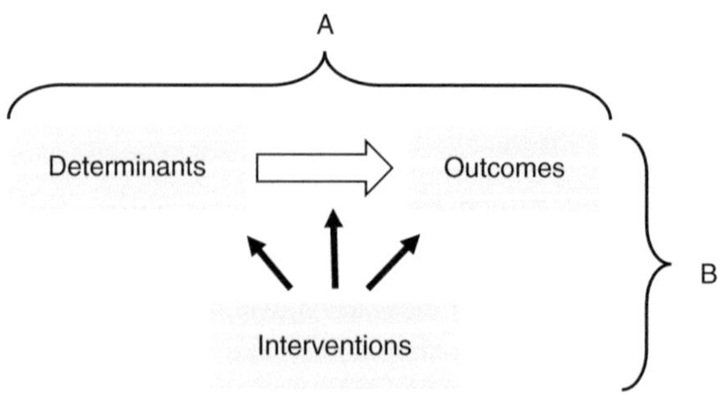

Fig. 1.3 Two dimensions of population health in which causal explanation plays a role: explanation of occurrence of determinants and outcomes (A) and explanation of success of interventions (B)

local data storage on desktop computers to repositories in the cloud. We believe that these transitions, which allow for ever faster data collection, curation, and analysis, deserve a robust framework for causal interpretation, or at least a framework that does not easily take the quality of inferences based on information that PHI provides for granted.

Slight Change of Scenery

While access to health information has become easier over time, the *interpretation* of information has received less attention. This theory-practice-gap is both a main motivation for, and the starting point of our discussion.

Causal explanation as an area of inquiry is part of philosophy of science. The *metaphysical* (What is causation? See Chap. 3.) and *epistemological* questions (How can we build causal knowledge? See Chap. 4.) have kept philosophers busy for centuries. The most prominent among them are probably Gottfried Wilhelm Leibniz (1646–1716), David Hume (1711–1776), Immanuel Kant (1724–1804), and John Stuart Mill (1806–1873). More recent work includes Mario Bunge's *Causality and Modern Science* (1959) [8], David Lewis' *Causation* (1973) [9], J.L. Mackie's *Cement of the Universe* (1974) [10], Wesley Salmon's *Scientific Explanation and the Causal Structure of the World* (1984) [11], Ellery Eells' *Probabilistic Causality* (1991) [12], Phil Dowe's *Physical Causation* (2000) [13], and Nancy Cartwright's *Hunting Causes and Using Them*[14], to name only a few selected examples. Each one of these thinkers has looked at the phenomenon of causation from a different angle, has proposed ways to define it, and has tried to outline ways to help you identify a cause if you find one. As so often in philosophy, there is no one solution to the problem. We believe that a concise, targeted discussion of some of these different approaches to causation might help those who work in PHI to make data gathering, management, analysis, and interpretation more interesting and perhaps even more fruitful.

This book surveys issues related to work that involves data, information, and knowledge management by taking a somewhat unusual approach. We integrate concepts and strategies from philosophy and informatics. We bring together views and arguments from philosophy of science with concepts from health information science in general, and from PHI in particular, with the hope that such interdisciplinary approach will contribute to improved population health by improving the theoretical underpinnings of the PHI endeavor.

At first glance, the two fields seem to have very little in common. By its very nature, philosophy of causation is a theoretical field and PHI is an applied science.[3] This is precisely why we propose to bring them together. We know of only one previous display of this unique ensemble of causation and PHI, reproduced here as Fig. 1.4, borrowed from [16:492]. The diagram depicts the feedback loop between the causal web of health-related phenomena in populations, the information systems that produce knowledge from health data, the policies and programs that are designed based on that knowledge, and the decisions and interventions; in short: the

[3] If it is a science at all. See, for example, Eden's discussion of the multiple paradigms of computer science (CS) that conceive of it as a branch of mathematics, engineering, or science [15].

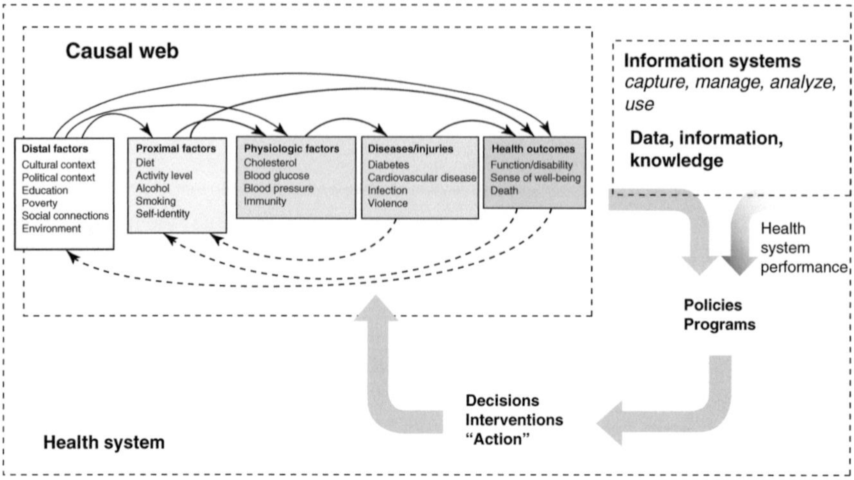

Fig. 1.4 Three critical systems in public health informatics: causation, policy, action. (Reprinted with permission from Tolentino et al. [16])

action that is justified by such policies and programs. We will discuss the fine points of these relationships later. At this point, it may suffice to say that this entire book can be seen as a commentary on Fig. 1.4 and, indeed, on the two currently available books on PHI [1] and PopHI [2].

Health data science is about generating useful information from health data in order to gather evidence that justifies knowledge for action. Thus, it is paramount to ensure that the interpretation of health data science results as evidence, and the effective use of knowledge for health decision-making, can – taken together – justify the intervention. It is precisely this goal of health data science, making a meaningful contribution to the effective improvement of a health care or prevention process, that asks for a causal explanation of such process. To identify risk factors and to put them in relation to one another *just is* to propose a causal explanation.

After data are defined and collected they are used to generate information, which in turn can be transformed into reliable knowledge. If this knowledge is good (and we will propose a few benchmarks for what "good" means in Chap. 6), subsequent medical and public health initiatives that target those risk factors are justified.

1.2 Etiology: Risk and Causation

The quest for understanding illness causation has a long history. We deliberately refrain from offering a historical survey; this has already been done by Alfred Evans [17] and Kay Codell Carter [18]. The causal thinking about a certain illness obviously changes over time according to the current status of scientific knowledge in a certain era. For example, different perceptions of stomach ulcer causation led to therapy with stress reduction and milk in the 1950s, acid-blockers in the 1970s, and antibiotics in the 1990's [19:3]. The underlying theoretical framework of assumptions gives rise to the overall paradigm of reasoning about illness causation, which has consequences for both medical and public health research.

Today's biomedical scientists work in either one of two broad scientific fields, epidemiology or laboratory science. Very few speak the language of both communities. Those working in patient care often speak neither of the two languages, sometimes one, and rarely both. Knowledge about illness causation is generated in these two fields by telling one of the following two stories.

Biochemical causation mechanisms are studied at the cellular and tissue micro-level. This part of the natural history of illness is called pathogenesis and this is the story told by basic scientists who work in laboratories and gain their knowledge by using experimental tools. Others will tell the story of natural history of illness in the language of risk, risk factors, and relative risk. This is the story told by epidemiologists, who study the occurrence of health phenomena by gathering data in populations and report their results at the macro level as aggregate information.

The person is the unit of observation in clinical medicine and the natural history of the disease of this person is described in detail in the medical chart of each individual patient. However, in order to draw any conclusions about the potential diagnosis, treatments, and prognosis, aggregate data from large populations are needed to verify that such conclusions are generally in sync with the natural history of disease in populations.

Those interested in the etiology of illness (defined as a disease, injury, or defect [20]) have two practical goals. First, they look for specific etiologic factors that can be singled out and offered to their colleagues in public health as targets for intervention. Second, they also try to understand the pathogenetic mechanisms underlying the process of becoming ill, in order to design interventions. There is a huge conceptual difference between these two goals, between the singling out of the worthy target for prevention initiatives and the understanding of what might be called the etiologic "process", which includes the pathogenetic mechanisms [21]. Epidemiologists can very well make (and already have made) an enormous contribution to both goals. However, their contribution towards the former might be considerably bigger than their contribution to the latter, where contributions from multiple disciplines are required for the elucidation of a complex etiologic process via the characterization of its component mechanisms.

Etiology is the story of illness occurrence and epidemiology is "disease occurrence research" [22]. Most etiology research is based on epidemiologic methodology, which enables us to study health and disease determinants in populations. Modern epidemiology [23] has moved far beyond the estimation of regional disease prevalence and outbreak research. It includes molecular [24] and genetic [25] aspects, one of the most recent additions is genomic epidemiology [26]. In almost every discipline of health research, epidemiologic methodology helps generate data that clarify etiologic and therapeutic aspects of health and disease.[4]

One of the goals of epidemiologists is, thus, to discover factors that are associated with changes in disease occurrence in populations. These factors, sometimes called *risk factors*, might be either protective or risk increasing. The predominant approach used to identify risk factors of disease is the design and conduct of research projects, in which epidemiologists observe groups of individuals. In one of the simplest cases, dividing the number of individuals with a disease by the total number of individuals in that group yields the *point prevalence* of disease in this population. The resulting percentage is interpreted as the prior (or: unconditional) probability of randomly choosing a diseased individual from that population. The point prevalence is an estimate of the magnitude of disease burden in defined populations at specific points in time.

In epidemiology, the issues of risk and causation are closely related. Causation is what epidemiologists try to identify, while risk is what they quantify when describing risk factors, which are associated with an increased likelihood of outcome occurrence. Neither one is easily defined. We think that the two are intertwined because they are two perspectives on the same process. In essence, we hold that risk and causation are two ways of looking at etiology, the process of illness occurrence. While the term *risk* is often used to frame the etiological process as a futuristic concept, *causation* is often used to tell the story by referring from some illness back to its causes. We will come back to this theme in Chap. 6.

1.3 Causal Theory in Epidemiology

Epidemiologists are interested in identifying causal relationships between certain exposures and illnesses [28]. They have been immensely successful in helping prevent illness and improve health. One major reason for this is that they have contributed to an increased understanding of causal relationships by developing an elaborate methodology to study the association between risk factors and illness in populations.

At least in part, this success is due to a continuing growth of a literature generated by theoreticians of epidemiology, who debate the mere concept of illness causation and the difficulties to identify causes [29–61]. Perhaps, this continued struggle might be fuelled by the fact that definitions of *cause* are manifold [62, 63] and perhaps impossible to be distilled into one single framework suitable for etiologic research.

It is quite impossible to summarize this literature in a few sentences, let alone to come up with a consensus on what constitutes a cause of illness and how it can be

[4]The most comprehensive textbooks about the theoretical underpinnings and inferential finepoints of epidemiology are Theoretical Epidemiology [22], Modern Epidemiology [23, 27], and Interpreting Epidemiologic Evidence [28].

identified using epidemiological research methodology. One difficulty is our apparent inability to agree on what we mean when we talk about causation; another is the difficulty to extract causal information from observational data based on set criteria.

The epidemiologic literature offers a variety of perspectives on causation. Perhaps the most important authors in this field are Mervyn Susser [38, 64], Ken Rothman [33], Douglas Weed [36, 61, 65], Sander Greenland [46, 52, 53, 66, 67] and Miguel Hernan/James Robins [56, 60].

Unfortunately, surprisingly little of what has been written by philosophers like Lewis [9], Mackie [10], Salmon [11, 68, 69], and Woodward [70, 71], to name only a few, is being received in epidemiology. Most recently, interest in causality in the health sciences has been rejuvenated by Jon Williamson and colleagues with an eye towards mechanism and evidence [63, 72–78] and by Alex Broadbent with a focus on explanation [79–81].

Indeed, the quest for a definition of illness causation in epidemiology has a very long history.[5] In his "Airs, waters, and places", Hippocrates offered a description of environmental and behavioral exposures one should consider when looking for health determinants:

> Whoever wishes to investigate medicine properly, should proceed thus: in the first place to consider the seasons of the year, and what effects each of them produces for they are not at all alike, but differ much from themselves in regard to their changes. Then the winds, the hot and the cold, especially such as are common to all countries, and then such as are peculiar to each locality. We must also consider the qualities of the waters, for as they differ from one another in taste and weight, so also do they differ much in their qualities. In the same manner, when one comes into a city to which he is a stranger, he ought to consider its situation, how it lies as to the winds and the rising of the sun; for its influence is not the same whether it lies to the north or the south, to the rising or to the setting sun. These things one ought to consider most attentively, and concerning the waters which the inhabitants use, whether they be marshy and soft, or hard, and running from elevated and rocky situations, and then if saltish and unfit for cooking; and the ground, whether it be naked and deficient in water, or wooded and well watered, and whether it lies in a hollow, confined situation, or is elevated and cold; and the mode in which the inhabitants live, and what are their pursuits, whether they are fond of drinking and eating to excess, and given to indolence, or are fond of exercise and labor, and not given to excess in eating and drinking.[6]

The history of epidemiology is full of most interesting examples of how vigilant observers like Hippocrates became smart investigators and helped develop the epidemiological approach to causation. Consider the following two examples.

Ignaz Semmelweis (1818–1865) observed that maternal childbed fever was much more frequent in a Viennese delivery ward that was served by students and doctors who had worked in the hospital morgue than in a delivery ward served by medical personnel who had not worked with cadavers right before the delivery. Semmelweis inferred, without knowing the mechanism, that handwashing might help. It did [82].

---

[5] Again, see the works by Alfred Evans [17] and Kay Codell Carter [18] for historical surveys.

[6] http://classics.mit.edu/Hippocrates/airwatpl.mb.txt; transl. Francis Adams

Another widely appreciated illustration is the London cholera outbreak (1854), which is mentioned in every introductory lecture on modern epidemiology. John Snow identified different sources of water supplied to different London neighborhoods as being associated with different cholera incidence rates. Snow carefully mapped these and brought his findings to the attention of local authorities with the suggestion to intervene. The legendary removal of the handle of the Broad Street water pump, although probably removed by authorities only after the epidemic had already started to decline [83], was nevertheless interpreted as proof that Snow was right [84]. This story serves as an illustration of the one-pathogen-one-disease paradigm of early infectious disease research.

The idea that "illnesses are best understood and controlled by focusing on their causes" [85] is usually attributed to Robert Koch (1843–1910) and has been called "the etiological standpoint" [18]. At the time, the much celebrated Henle-Koch postulates were indeed a breakthrough in etiologic theory [86], claiming that a single agent always causes the same disease, and the same disease is always being caused by this very agent. In infectious disease research, this single cause view still plays a central role, for example in discussions of HIV as the cause of AIDS [87]. It is also an example of manipulationist counterfactual reasoning in illness causation research.[7] Note that both Semmelweis and Snow lived and worked long before bacteriology began to offer biological explanations for their observations.

Perhaps the most likely reason for the continued success of the strong connectionist view of illness causation is the idea that only necessary causes are causes of illness. The idea that some causes might be necessary, but not sufficient to initiate disease, is less widely accepted. In this case, one would expect the infectious agent to be present in most, even all cases of disease, but it might also be present in individuals without the disease. This is the case in longterm-survivors of HIV infection who do not seroconvert for many years [88], who can be viewed as the Popperian black swans that help refute the conjecture that all swans are white; an example that was discussed in the epidemiological literature a few decades ago [89, 90].

The current tendency is to de-emphasize single causes [91] in favor of causal complexes [39], constellations [33], pathways [92], or webs [41], which unfortunately often remain unexplained, leaving it unclear how they are epistemologically constrained [70:22/23]. Even genetic causation seems to be much more complex than previously assumed and researchers now acknowledge that there is no perfect 1:1 relationship between a particular mutation and disease occurrence [58]. One extreme position is that causation cannot be seen, proven, or even be made certain, because it is an expert's judgment, not a natural phenomenon to be discovered [61].

One crucial aspect of the idea that illness has specific identifiable causes is that avoiding them reduces the likelihood of illness occurrence. Our motivation here is that despite the recognition of multifactorial disease models in the medical and lay communities, current etiologic research is still dominated by attempts to identify *independent* risk factors, i.e., presumably causal antecedents of illness that contribute to illness occurrence independent of others. Such independent risk factors are

[7] See Chap. 3 for details on the concept of counterfactual causation.

usually characteristics present in an appreciably larger proportion of cases (individuals with the illness) than controls (those without the illness under investigation), thus being statistically associated with the illness while adjusting for potential confounders. However, the current conception of multifactorial causes holds that

> all kinds of causal factors form a 'causal complex', 'causal web' or 'web of causation' that contributes to the development of a disease. Each factor is neither necessary nor sufficient, for producing the disease state, but their combination and potentiation lead to the effect [58]

This apparent disconnect – a focus on preventable risk factors despite our acknowledgment that there is often no such thing as a single necessary cause of illness – deserves consideration.

One response to these complexities comes from Phillippe and Mansi, who attempt to introduce the notion of non-linear dynamics into epidemiology. They see epidemiology as a mainly linear approach that does "not account explicitly for structural nonlinearity" [45]. Coming from infectious disease epidemiology, where outcomes are not independent of each other since inter-personal contact is needed for infection [93], the authors suggest taking disease occurrence as *emergence*, as unpredictable, unexpected and unexplained, and fractality as an organization pattern with structural similarity across a hierarchy of several scales. Implicitly, they suggest replacing Humean strong connectionism with a non-linear, probabilistic model of disease causation. Phillippe and Mansi's suggestion is supplemented by probabilistic approaches to causation, such as those put forward by Reichenbach, Good, Suppes, Eells, Hitchcock and other non-deterministic philosophers of causality.[8] However, the practical suggestion by Phillippe and Mansi that neural network-based analytic techniques might be better in predicting outcomes than, e.g., logistic regression approaches has not found much support in epidemiology.

The classic concept of epidemiological thinking about causation was put forward by Ken Rothman in 1976 [33]. The idea is that it always takes multiple component causes for disease occurrence, and that necessary and sufficient causes should not be considered at the same explanatory level. Sufficient causal constellations (depicted in figures as "pies") are composed of units (pieces of the pies called "component causes") that are either necessary, i.e., present in all sufficient causal constellations, or non-necessary, i.e., present in some, but not all causal constellations.[9]

This model has, to our knowledge, been revised [95], but not modified. Aspects of it had previously been discussed by Susser [64], who later [38] traced the concept of necessary and sufficient causes back to Galileo, via Bunge, who quotes Il Saggiatore (1623), [8:33].

Probably the most challenging question is the impossibility-of-scientific-proof conundrum. Rothman and Greenland [95] hold that per Hume, proof cannot be achieved in science because at both the experimental and epidemiologic levels only association, but not causation can be observed [95:22]: "Even the most careful and detailed mechanistic dissection of individual events cannot provide more than

[8] See, e.g., [94] for an excellent recent collection of essays.

[9] See Chap. 3 for details.

associations, albeit at a finer level". Even at this finer level, the problem persists that not all X are always followed by Y, which suggests two possible world views: either, the world is deterministic and our observation techniques and/or levels of observation do not allow for an appropriate perception of strong (deterministic) causal connections, or the world is indeterministic, "meaning that there are particular events which lack a sufficient cause" [94:1]. This probabilistic model of component causes, however, still needs to be developed in a fashion that further clarifies the suggested dose-response relationship between components of causal constellations and the likelihood of disease occurrence. The fact that most philosophers who discuss probabilistic causation select examples from disease occurrence (e.g., smoking and lung cancer [12]) not only suggest that examples from disease causation are good examples for discussions of probabilistic causation, but also that probabilistic models of causation are a good fit for discussions of disease occurrence. In theory, researchers may wish to fix the deterministic problem of Rothman's pies by "simply think(ing) of the components as contributing together to the probability of the effect, rather than being sufficient for it" [50]. In practice, all epidemiologists can provide is an approximation of "real" causes via the identification of risk factors.

1.4 Kantian Lament

Aristotle's famous first statement in his Metaphysics that "all men by nature desire to know" may well be the driving force behind our desire to extract causal knowledge from observed data structures. However, this might be doomed to failure since it uses the Plato-Cartesian dualism of surface data associations versus underlying causal structure, which leads us to the all-too-familiar notion that "association can never prove causation" [96]. If we define observed data as insufficient for causal inference, we cannot identify causation from observed data.

In his 1991 article *What is a cause and how do we know one?*, Mervyn Susser used the subtitle *A grammar for pragmatic epidemiology*. Using this as a point of departure, we argue that many problems in current disease causation thinking just *cannot* be resolved. If we agree that absolute proof is impossible in science, that correlation may not be causation, and that even experimental evidence of output changes after input manipulation does not suffice to establish causation indubitably, causation might be impossible to establish.

This is what Richard Rorty has called the *Kantian lament*, the notion "that we are forever trapped behind the veil of subjectivity", the "pointless, because tautologous, claim that something we define as being beyond our knowledge is, alas, beyond our knowledge" [97:58]. If we carried Susser's pragmatic grammar to the next level by embracing a neo-pragmatic approach to disease causation, we should abandon definitions of causation that rely on concepts such as truth, in favor of conceptions of causation that have in mind solely the improvement of the human condition by minimization of suffering.[10]

The Henle-Koch view of individual causes leading to individual diseases has led to the concept of causal inference by criteria, such as those put forward by Sir Austin Bradford Hill [32], probably developed with Hume's help [99]. Unfortunately, the postulation of criteria such as Hill's, Susser's [34, 38], and our own [100], is a mere replacement of one dilemma with another. Why should it be easier to identify the truth condition of the criteria than identifying the true relationship between exposures and their effects that develops before our very eyes? In fact, the very idea to develop criteria for causal inference does not seem pragmatic at all. The pragmatist would ask, how can we identify causes in a way that makes our lives a little better? Since there is not much room for absolute reference in pragmatism either, the identification of causation does not make much sense beyond enabling us to act upon them in order to improve the human condition. Indeed, without absolute reference, the entire concept of verification, and, for that matter, falsification [101], seems difficult beyond the comparison of criteria to gold standards, which are notoriously soft in nature and can be misleading if incorrect [102]. The very notion of criteria encapsulates the view of *if, and only if*, which is deterministic lingo and concept *par excellence* and, therefore, does not fit probabilistic notions of illness causation too well.

1.5 What This Book Is, and Is Not About

First of all, this book is about causal explanation in the context of PHI, not an overview of public health informatics or population health informatics.[11]

Second, the book does not provide a general introduction to the philosophy of science, nor to the philosophy of causation in particular. Indeed, we do not intend it to be a "philosophy book" at all. We deal with only one component of all philosophy of science, causation, and even that sub-field is too wide and too deep to be covered in a way that does justice to all its intricacies that would deserve attention. The interested reader is referred to the Oxford Handbook of Causation [103] and "Causation in the Sciences" [104]; both offer an overarching and multifaceted treatment of the topic. Also, the online Stanford Encyclopedia of Philosophy (plato.

---

[10] Perhaps, the attempt to prove causation is not only misleading because of some epidemiologic version of the Kantian lament, but also because the cause is sometimes a cause *and also* a characteristic of the disease under investigation. See Mumford and Anjum's dispositionalist account, discussed in Chap. 3, for an interesting take on this possibility [98].

[11] Such overviews have been provided by Magnuson and Fu [1] and by Joshi, Thorpe, and Waldron [2].

stanford.edu) is an outstanding and free resource that will be helpful to all readers who are eager to dive a bit deeper into the philosophy of causation.

Third, this is not a guide to causal *inference* in public health. The title of Susser's paper "What is a cause and how do we know one?" [38] suggests that answers are possible. Indeed, some authors in public health information science support this notion by writing that

> To establish the cause-and-effect relationship, five criteria must be present: strength of association (the association must be clear), consistency (observation of the association must be repeatable in different populations at different times), temporality (the cause must precede the effect), plausibility (the explanation must make sense biologically), and biological gradient (there must be a dose–response relationship) [105]

As discussed above, clear-cut causal inference like this is impossible. We do not have the space, nor the goal, in this book to discuss this issue at full length. This has been done elsewhere, i.e., in numerous articles on "criteria" for causation in the health sciences, especially the viewpoints proposed by occupational epidemiologist Sir Austin Bradford Hill [32]. We refer the interested reader to papers by Alfredo Morabia [99, 106], John Ioannidis [107], and one of us [108].

Fourth, and perhaps most importantly, this book is not intended to offer an exhaustive answer to the question, What role does causal explanation play in Public Health Informatics? A comprehensive answer to that question needs more exploration than is possible in this book. A broader discussion is needed before we and others can take a serious stab at answers. Consider this book an attempt to find a way to open that can; we will deal with the worms later.

1.6 Overview of Chapters

Here is a brief overview of the chapters to follow. Chapter 2 will introduce our framework, *health data science,* and discuss its technical, mathematical-conceptual, and reasoning components. In Chap. 3 we discuss the metaphysics of causation and in Chap. 4 we give an overview of its epistemological aspects. Chapter 5 is on making knowledge for population health. We briefly review the main current framework of knowledge generation from data via information and offer our own version. In Chap. 6 we survey the concepts of individual and population risk, give examples for univariable and multivariable risk estimation, and suggest that risk estimation is causal explanation at the population level. Chapter 7 turns toward evidence integration, and Chap. 8 concludes and invites your input and feedback.

Chapter 2
Health Data Science

Abstract In this chapter, we introduce the concept of Health Data Science and define its three domains: technology, analytics, and conceptual. In the technology domain, we drill down from computer science via health informatics to public health informatics. The analytics domain includes biostatistics, bioinformatics, epidemiology, and simulation. In the conceptual domain, we introduce the philosophy of information, and of health and causation. Taken together, these domains provide the theoretical backdrop for the remainder of the book.

Keywords Technology · Analytics · Concept · Informatics · Biostatistics Epidemiology · Information · Philosophy

2.1 Data Science

Data Science has emerged as

Definition A new transdisciplinary field that builds on and synthesizes a number of relevant disciplines and bodies of knowledge, including statistics, informatics, computing, communication, management, and sociology, to study data following 'data science thinking' [109].

This definition, written by Longbing Cao, Professor in the Advanced Analytics Institute at the University of Technology Sydney, Australia, envisions data science to integrate data from a certain domain using 'data science thinking'. What is unique about his proposal is that he makes explicit the intellectual challenge that comes with this new field. Cao thinks that "data scientists aim to invent data and intelligence-driven machines to represent, learn, simulate, reinforce, and transfer human-like intuition, imagination, curiosity, and creative thinking through human-data interaction and cooperation" [109:59]. With this book, we'd like to make a contribution to the "*thinking*" part. Indeed, we consider that thinking about causation and causal explanation is at the epicenter of health data science. In keeping with this perspective, Lucila Ohno-Machado, Editor-in-Chief of the Journal of the American Medical Informatics Association (JAMIA), holds that the main characteristics of (biomedical)

O. Dammann, B. Smart, *Causation in Population Health Informatics and Data Science*, https://doi.org/10.1007/978-3-319-96307-5_2

data science are the goal to promote health and the method that allows us to "alleviate the burden of disease through clever transformation of data into knowledge" [110].

The information turn[1] in general, and biomedical health informatics in particular, have revolutionized the ways we deal with health data and manufacture knowledge in helpful ways. Examples are the electronic medical record (EMR) in medical care, electronic surveillance systems in public health informatics, and risk analysis methodologies in epidemiology.

Our working definition of *Health Data Science* (HDS) for the purpose of this book is:

Definition *Health Data Science* is scientific work performed to improve the collection, management, and analysis of health-related data from individuals or populations, with the goal to improve their health.

In this sense, HDS methodology has at least three large and overlapping components (Fig. 2.1):

1. A *technological* component, including health informatics and computer science aspects;
2. An *analytical* component, including biostatistics, bioinformatics, epidemiology, and simulation;

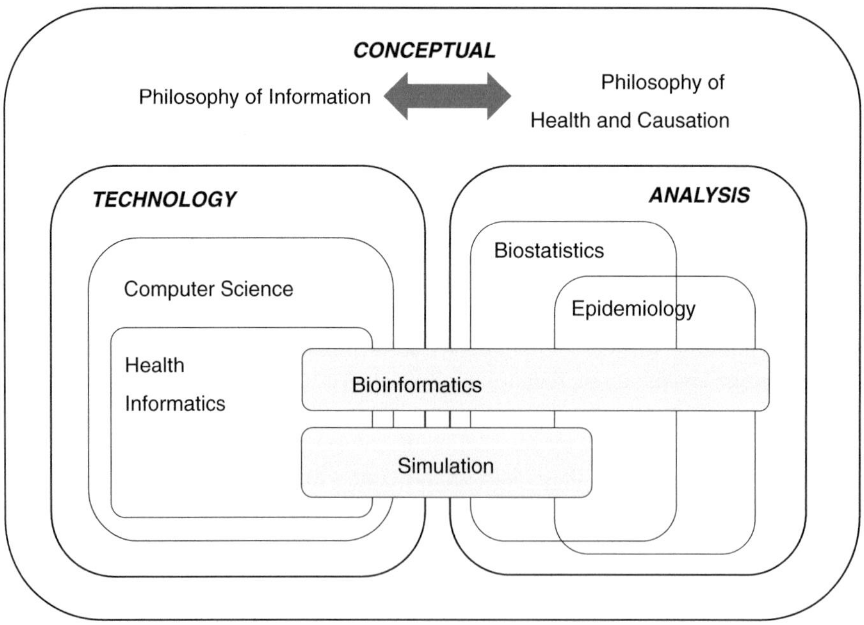

Fig. 2.1 Domains of health data science

[1]The term "information turn" was probably coined by Luciano Floridi [111], describing what he "defined as the fourth revolution in our self-understanding, after the Copernican, the Darwinian, and the Freudian ones"[112:3].

3. A *conceptual-reasoning* component that comprises two large fields in modern philosophy, philosophy of information and philosophy of health and causation.

Note that these domains are neither collectively exhaustive, nor mutually exclusive. We consider all components to refer mainly to their biomedical/health aspects of informatics and information science. Moreover, the schema in Fig. 2.1 keeps theoretically separate what is closely related in practice. In the remainder of this chapter, we devote one section to each domain.

2.2 The Technology Domain

2.2.1 Computer Science

The Technology Domain is, put simply, *computer science* applied to health improvement in medicine and public health.

It is not trivial to define computer science. For our present purpose, we use the following definition:

Definition *Computer science* is the professional concern with the design, analysis, and maintenance of software and hardware systems.

Although this is a rather broad definition, we think it makes an important point. Computer science really encompasses all things computer from the design and construction of physical hardware to algorithms and all kinds of software. We have training "comp sci" programs and departments at colleges and universities, as well as companies that perform computer science in all shapes and colors.

From the perspective we take in this book, the philosophy of computer science is of interest because it concerns theoretical aspects of computer science, among other issues.[2] Computer science is, broadly speaking, considered a discipline of mathematics, engineering, and/or a scientific discipline [15]. The last perspective is of particular importance to our topic, because we come from the population health data science perspective. Any data science is rooted in the principles of computation and depends on developments in computer science. If health data science is an interdisciplinary effort to improve health, computer science and computation *as* a science should be considered part of that interdisciplinary effort to improve health. We concur with Matti Tedre, who argues that computer science is an empirical science in that it uses scientific methods of data gathering, hypothesis testing, and inference based on results [113]. It is that inferential realm where we hope our discussion will make a contribution, because causal explanation has so far been neglected in the philosophy of computation.

---

[2] See Turner, Raymond and Angius, Nicola, "The Philosophy of Computer Science", The Stanford Encyclopedia of Philosophy (Spring 2017 Edition), Edward N. Zalta (ed.), URL = <https://plato.stanford.edu/archives/spr2017/entries/computer-science/>.

2.2.2 Health Informatics

We adapt the following definition of *informatics* as

Definition Computer science in specific practical or theoretical contexts.

According to this definition, the field of informatics is rather broad and includes computer science, software engineering, as well as information systems and technology. Although it is, in this sense, a rather theoretical field, it is pursued with a practical goal, because it provides responses to certain organizational needs.

Medical informatics started in the 1960s and '70s as a discipline for mathematicians and computer scientists who moved into medicine to support hospitals that were often caught off guard by the immense progress during those years in terms of hardware development and availability outside academia. But even today it is still considered a young discipline [114].

One generalized view of health informatics (HIMSS, 2014) holds that

Definition *Health informatics* is the interdisciplinary study of the design, development, adoption, and application of IT-based innovations in healthcare services delivery, management, and planning.

In the context of health information science, however, we need to consider research activities that utilize informatics tools to improve the health of individuals and populations.

Thus, we define "health science informatics" as follows:

Definition *Health Science Informatics* is any utilization of informatics tools and methods in health science activities designed to contribute to better health for individuals and populations.

Health science informatics provides the tools for data collection and generation in the health sciences, be it experimental research in small systems such as cell-cultures, or in large scale epidemiological studies.

2.2.3 Public Health Informatics

Public Health Informatics (PHI) is the computational toolbox for the public health researcher, administrator, field worker, and interventionist [1, 2]. Four areas of particular importance for PHI are (1) health promotion in populations, (2) disease prevention by risk alteration, (3) exploration of the potential for prevention at all vulnerable points in the causal chains, and (4) reflection of the governmental context of public health practice [1:11].

Most recently, Dixon and coworkers [115] suggested a conceptual framework in which the "Essential Services" in public health (assessment, policy development, and assurance) are based on three layers that consist of ethics, a socio-technical informatics infrastructure and, at the very bottom, research, workforce development and financial support. From this model it follows that any PHI application should be practice-oriented in that it should be designed to support the specific activity in each Essential Service in public health. In order to be helpful in practice, however, surveillance data and epidemiological research results need to be integrated. Because public health practice is to a large extent focused on interventions (such as immunizations, health behavior modifications, and policies), much of the evidence needed to justify such interventions is related to the causal processes that) generate the population health problem to be prevented.

Public health actions need to be based on solid and timely population data [116]. The major data-generating disciplines in public health are surveillance, research, and evaluation. Their common denominator is computational data management and analysis. Therefore, all three are heavily, if not mainly, informatics-based methods [117].

2.2.3.1 Surveillance

Public health surveillance (PHS) is the "systematic and continuous collection, analysis, and interpretation of data, closely integrated with the timely and coherent dissemination of the results and assessment to those who have the right to know so that action can be taken" [118]. Public Health Surveillance) is an evolving, complex and rather heterogeneous area of informatics application [119]. Still, the main task of PHS is straightforward: "It should provide information to the public health community regarding the health of the populations served" [120].

Public Health Surveillance data are mainly data about the prevalence and incidence of certain diseases or injuries, their severity and impact [121:19]. Major data sources are health surveys, registries, health records, environmental monitoring, research and other sources, such as census data or criminal justice information [122:6]. The five main domains of PHS are system development and data collection, data management and information integration, data analysis and interpretation), communication of findings, and evaluation of the surveillance system [123:viii]. Unfortunately, the literature on analysis and interpretation of public health surveillance data is silent when it comes to causal explanation of observed phenomena. Can public health surveillance data be "used to detect epidemics, …, evaluate prevention programs, and project future public health needs" [124:88] without theoretical guidance on how to interpret observed data as valid evidence in support of causal claims?

2.2.3.2 Research

Although some have called epidemiology *the basic science of public health* [125:350–2], "public health is far more complex than merely applying epidemiology" [126]. Still, much of public health research is performed in epidemiology, the study of the distribution and determinants of disease frequency in human [127] or animal populations [128].

Epidemiological analyses that include the measurement of molecular [24] and genomic data [26] can sometimes deliver data about observed associations that are usually reserved for laboratory experiments. However, the optimistic prospect of improved medicine and public health via more detailed molecular data gathering is likely to fail because "many, if not most biomolecular mechanisms that translate the human genomic information into phenotypes are not known yet and, thus, most of the molecular and cellular data collected will not lead to biomedically relevant conclusions" [129].

Epidemiologists design studies to elucidate the etiology of diseases by calculating measures of association between certain risk factors and specified health outcomes in well-defined populations. The result is often an estimate of the relative risk, i.e., the risk of developing a specific outcome given exposure, divided by the risk among those not so exposed. However, one of the main problems in epidemiology, just as in surveillance, is to find causal relationships in the observed data [50, 130]. Philosopher Alex Broadbent has recently called this the "causal interpretation problem": the mathematical definition of the above measures of association does not contain an extra ingredient that would help us "understand the causal import of a measure of association [...] when it is used to express a causal fact, as well as a fact about an association" [80:30].

2.2.3.3 Evidence-Based Medicine

The Scottish epidemiologist Archie Cochrane pioneered evidence-based medicine (EBM) through his book *Effectiveness and Efficiency: Random Reflections on Health Services* [131] and subsequent advocacy. In 1992 the evidence-based medicine working group proposed EBM as a new approach to teaching the practice of medicine [132]. A group of Canadian researchers defined EBM as "the conscientious, explicit, and judicious use of current best evidence in making decisions about the care of individual patients" [133]. EBM aims to integrate clinical expertise with the techniques from a variety of scientific and technical fields, such as systematic access to medical literature), risk-benefit analysis, and clinical epidemiology. EBM applies the best available evidence gained from the scientific method to clinical decision making [134].

2.2.3.4 Evaluation

The Centers for Disease Control and Prevention provides a comprehensive Framework for Program Evaluation in Public Health [135]. The first three steps are preparatory: include all stakeholders, provide a good description of the program, and focus on evaluation design. Steps 4 and 5 are about data collection (gather credible evidence) and analysis (justify conclusions). Causal inference can help find out whether the evidence is credible and whether conclusions are justified.

2.3 The Analytics Domain

2.3.1 *Biostatistics*

Statistical approaches employed in the life sciences are called *biostatistics*. The biostatistical toolbox contains methods that allow investigators to summarize certain characteristics of datasets and the variables they contain, such as frequency distributions, means and standard deviations, among others. This part of biostatistics is called *descriptive* biostatistics, because it provides descriptions of variables in the form of summary measures, which are needed to compare one dataset with another. Another part is *inferential* biostatistics, which includes pertinent techniques needed to analyze datasets in comparison to one another in order to test hypotheses.

At this point, biostatistics intersects with causal reasoning. For example, two groups of individuals that differ in one and only one outcome characteristic are compared, e.g., cutaneous melanoma present (group A) versus absent (group B). It turns out that individuals in group A are twice as likely to have a history of more than ten severe sunburns compared to members of group B [136]. To exclude the possibility that this is a chance finding, we need assurance that the two are unlikely to come from the same underlying population. To do this, a particular statistical test is applied to the data that provides an estimate of the likelihood that we are wrong in assuming that the two sets do not come from the same underlying probability distribution (alternative hypothesis) although they actually do (*null hypothesis*). By convention, this probability measure (p) is taken to give reasonable assurance when it turns out to be less than 5% ($p < 0.05$).

The intersection with causal reasoning pertains to the question whether this difference in exposure to sunlight is responsible for the differential in melanoma risk. We will come back to *risk* in Chap. 6.

2.3.2 *Bioinformatics*

Coined by Paulien Hogeweg in 1970, the meaning of the term "bioinformatics" has evolved in parallel with the development of laboratory science over the past half century. Today, the term is used to comprise computational data analysis methods that allow us to "make sense" of data from biological samples. These data are frequently so-called "omics" data, i.e., data that reveal the entire genome (genomics) or all proteins (proteomics) in a sample.

The current and expected future roles for bioinformatics so defined in causal reasoning in medicine and public health is often wildly overstated or misguided. For example, in a paper entitled "On deducing causality in metabolic networks", Bodei and colleagues write that

> We exploit a reading of chemical reactions in terms of logical implications: starting from a description of a metabolic network in terms of reaction rules and initial conditions, chains of reactions, causally depending one from the another (sic), can be automatically deduced [137].

If the computer script, upon query, spits out causal relationships when input data appear to follow the pre-programmed rules for causal relationships, it remains to be discussed whether this is an entirely circular reasoning process and if it might be necessary to first feed the system causal information in order for it to provide causal inference (an example of what Cartwright has called "no causation in, no causation out" [138]).

Some bioinformatics tools of the future will undoubtedly make great contributions to improvements in health care. In particular, translational bioinformatics has become an area of research that links bioinformatics and healthcare [139].

Although data scientists are traditionally reluctant to make causal claims, at least some bioinformaticians appear to think otherwise:

> Holistic approaches, integrating data from several sources, e.g. genomic and epigenomic, will increase the understanding of the underlying biological concepts and provide *insight into the causes, effects and effective solutions.* ([140], emphasis ours).

Part of the motivation for this book stems from the recognition that the "providing insights" part of the above statement cannot do without the conceptual and reasoning components of health data science. The idea of better data integration as a promising future goal is ubiquitous in the health informatics literature, but cogent solutions how to accomplish that goal are hard to come by.

2.3.3 Epidemiology

The third part of the conceptual-mathematical component is the research field known as "epidemiology", and in our current context mainly the sub discipline sometimes called *risk factor epidemiology.*[3] In risk factor epidemiology, data of the best possible quality are collected from well-defined populations, such as all citizens of Johannesburg, or populations of study participants selected for a particular epidemiological study.

The main purpose of risk factor epidemiology is to identify in such populations factors that are associated with an increased or decreased risk for a specified health outcome. Achieving this goal requires a thoughtful study design, including the careful definition of study populations and the collection of reliable and valid data, among other things. These data are analyzed, often using biostatistical methods, according to the rules of epidemiological analysis design, which define exposure variables, outcome variables, and ask for the calculation of a measure of association and a measure of statistical significance, among other requirements that are not of

[3]The term is not used frequently in epidemiological practice. We use it here to distinguish it from all other kinds of epidemiology that do not focus on risk factor discovery.

primary importance here. To offer an example from the epidemiological work of one of us (O.D.), we found that the co-occurrence of bacteria and inflammation in the placenta of extremely preterm newborns (i.e., exposure to infection and inflammation before birth) was associated with an increased risk for retinopathy of prematurity in the center of the newborn's retina (i.e., outcome in newborns after birth). The risk was increased threefold (odds ratio, 3.1) and statistically significant (95% confidence interval, 1.02–9.5) [141].

There are many other requirements to be satisfied before such statistical associations are taken for granted as a measure of causal associations. We will go into such detail in Chap. 5.

2.3.4 Simulation

Last, but not least, simulation plays a growing and ever more important role as a method in the quantitative biosciences. While *risk factor epidemiology* is a bottom-up analysis of real-life data, *simulation* represents a top-down approach that allows scientists to try out their assumptions about the mechanism and function of a certain real-life phenomenon. Epidemiologists collect data and transform them into information to generate evidence that is eventually turned into knowledge by the community. Simulationists (an awkward term, but "simulators" sounds even worse) generate data and try to imitate the process of information-making and evidence generation. A combination of both approaches, enriched with network analyses of data, is what we have termed "systems epidemiology" [142].

2.4 The Conceptual Domain

2.4.1 Philosophy of Information

The beginning of the information age is considered *the third revolution*, following the agricultural and industrial revolutions. The ubiquitous availability of progressively more inexpensive and technologically more powerful computers has changed virtually all areas of human life.

In the footsteps of philosophy of computation and of philosophy of artificial intelligence, the philosophy of information came of age in 2011 with Luciano Floridi's book of the same title [112]. He sees philosophy of information as a "foundational philosophy of information-design and conceptual engineering" [112:25]. Floridi thinks that philosophy of information "promises to be one of the most exciting and fruitful areas of research of our time" (ibid). His excellent book provides strong support for this notion. Indeed, the book is probing deep into what he calls "the information turn" in philosophy (probably being intended to represent the next turn after the "linguistic turn" in philosophy; see [143]).

In our context, one particularly interesting area of inquiry is situated at the intersection of philosophy of information and causal relevance [112, Chap. 11]. Floridi makes this explicit in the section on epistemic vs. causal relevance. He follows Cohen's and Borlund's theories by distinguishing between system-oriented S-theories and agent-oriented A-theories of relevance, and he follows David Hitchcock in relating S-theories to causal relevance and A-theories to epistemic relevance.

We think that this distinction is rather important, because - as Floridi writes –

> S-theories usually analyse relevance in terms of [...] various forms of *conditional in/dependence* (how some information can help produce some outcome) [...] (while) A-theories tend to analyse relevance in terms of [...] perceived *utility, informativeness, beneficiality* and other ways of 'bearing on the matter at hand' in relation to an agent's informational needs (ibid., p.247).

Thus, in some sense, both S- and A-theories are interesting, but S-theories are more pertinent to our topic of causal reasoning in health data science, simply because issues related to conditional in/dependence are closer to the center of causal reasoning than issues related to the satisfaction of an agent's informational needs. For example, a relevant answer to the question of how certain information can be helpful in healthcare settings is more important to us (at least in this book) than a relevant answer to the question of how some agent's informational needs can be satisfied, because finding an answer to the former question requires direct causal reasoning at the system level, while finding an answer to the latter requires smart solution-finding in terms of fast and efficient information retrieval and logistics at the agent level, be it a single health information scientist, her entire research team, or a large research institute affiliated with a national network of hospitals. Our focus in this book is not on philosophy of information but on philosophy of causation, the topic of the next section as well as Chaps. 3 and 4.

2.4.2 *Philosophy of Health and Causation*

In health data science, causation research began its career as a central topic in biostatistics and epidemiology sometime during the second half of the twentieth century. The two most important interrelated issues in our current context are causal inference and causal explanation. During the same timeframe, philosophy of causation had some sort of comeback; Mackie, Bunge, Salmon, Eels, Sosa, Dowe, Woodward, Cartwright, Mumford and Anjum, Paul and Hall and Dupré, to mention only a few, have contributed to this renaissance of causation as a socially acceptable area of philosophical inquiry.

The next two chapters provide an introduction to conceptual issues related to causation, causal explanation, and causal inference in the health sciences. We will build on discussions from the recent philosophical literature. As we do not require readers to have prior knowledge of philosophy of causation, we want at least to share a few introductory comments here that may ease the transition from technology and analysis domains to our discussion of how causation is studied in contemporary philosophy, and where our project fits in.

Let us offer an example of how philosophy of causation and healthcare research practice are related. The analytic domain outlined in the previous section encompasses, in essence, methodologies that analyze data from observations in large groups of individuals.[4] In essence, a large number of individuals is classified according to pre-defined variables of interest. In risk factor epidemiology, for example, the target relationship of interest is the *exposure-outcome* relationship. In statistics, measures of association (of which correlation is a special case) quantify the strength of that association, whether causal or not.

Through the centuries, philosophers have wrestled with just that problem: that of finding justification to move from *association* to causation. This is what we mean when we talk about *causal inference*. The philosopher John Stuart Mill published his ideas about scientific reasoning and causal inference using the methods of scientific investigation in the second half of the nineteenth century. In his *System of Logic,* Mill touches upon multiple issues important to causal inference in the health sciences, e.g., the idea that our world seems to be non-deterministic in its causal structure [144:203] and that any phenomenon has not just one, but multiple antecedents (214). He devotes a long chapter to "Experimental Inquiry", motivated by his insight that "observation … without experiment … can ascertain sequences and co-existences, but cannot prove causation" (253).

In medicine and public health, a similar reliance is placed on intervention studies (observational and intervention studies can yield very different results). Here is a classic example. Meir Stampfer and co-authors pooled data from multiple prospective studies on the effect of hormone replacement therapy (HRT) to coronary heart disease (CHD) risk [145]. They inferred a relative reduction of nearly 50% with use of HRT and stated that "overall, the bulk of the evidence strongly supports a protective effect of estrogens that is unlikely to be explained by confounding factors". A randomized clinical trial was then carried out to evaluate the major health benefits and risks of HRT by comparing women with established CHD to healthy women. A different conclusion was reached: HRT was associated with slightly *increased* risk of CHD [146, 147]. It turned out that socioeconomic position was a confounding variable. When all measures of socioeconomic position across the life course were adjusted for, a slightly higher risk of CHD was associated with HRT use, consistent with the randomized trial results [148]. Another bias, the timing of HRT treatment in relation to menopause, was discussed as a likely culprit [149].

This is just one example how philosophy of causation and health research intersect. The next two chapters will provide a more detailed overview and discussion.

[4] We will go into more detail in Chap. 6.

2.5 Summary

In this chapter we have outlined the three domains of our framework for health data science, its technological, analytic, and conceptual components. We have offered a visual depiction of this framework in Fig. 2.1 that displays the relationship between the domains and their components as we see them. According to this framework, the technology domain comprises fields such as computer science, with health (or biomedical) informatics being the center of discussion. In the analysis domain, traditional data analysis techniques such as biostatistics, epidemiology, bioinformatics, and simulation cover overlapping areas. Some of them, e.g., bioinformatics and simulation, build bridges to the technological side of things. The third, conceptual domain, is composed of the philosophical approaches to information and causation in medicine/epidemiology, which provide overarching theoretical views of the other two components.

The next chapter will introduce to the metaphysics of illness causation.

Chapter 3
The Metaphysics of Illness Causation

Abstract In this chapter we provide a philosophical discussion of the nature of causation, as applied to the investigation of disease etiology and preventive and curative interventions. This chapter is primarily an exercise in metaphysics and conceptual analysis, in which we analyze existing concepts of causation dating back to David Hume's eighteenth century empiricism, right up to the public health-specific analysis provided by Kenneth Rothman, and the more recent dispositionalist ontologies of Stephen Mumford and Rani Lill Anjum. We argue that different metaphysical concepts of causation are implicit in different research methodologies in the medical sciences. We relate J. L. Mackie's "Inus condition" metaphysic of causation to Rothman's epidemiologic account of disease etiology, and go on to discuss "The counterfactual account of causation". The latter is often used by epidemiologists as an alternative nomenclature of the "potential outcomes approach" to causal inference. We will show why this is the case, and identify differences between this strategy for causal inference in public health and the popular philosophical view. We conclude that the concepts of causation employed in the health sciences are integral to their practice, whether used consciously or unconsciously, and that a clear insight into the nature of the metaphysical and conceptual schemes underlying the etiological process would help all those working in the medicine and public health.

Keywords Philosophy of disease · Regularity theory · Counterfactuals
Dispositionalism · Disease etiology

3.1 Introduction

The epidemiologist's primary goal is to apply systematic methodologies to gather knowledge about illness etiology, and to identify suitable interventions. Epidemiologists typically identify the etiology of an illness by conducting studies (such as observational studies and randomised controlled trials) on specified populations, and then systematically interpreting the data using a variety of statistical methods. As we mentioned in the previous chapter, some of the main difficulties faced by epidemiologists arise from a lack of agreement on a definition of "cause",

O. Dammann, B. Smart, *Causation in Population Health Informatics and Data Science*, https://doi.org/10.1007/978-3-319-96307-5_3

and the absence of criteria to *prove* a genuine causal relation between the exposure and outcome under investigation (as opposed to identifying mere associations).

In the following two chapters, we will address a number of metaphysical (this chapter) and epistemological problems (Chap. 4) concerning causes and causal inference in population health data science. In this chapter we outline several philosophical analyses of causation (some first advocated by philosophers as far back as the eighteenth century), and how they might guide us and help us understand epidemiological research. We save the second question for Chap. 4, in which we move from definitions of causation, to the practical problem of inferring causation in the medical sciences.

3.2 Illness Causation: Causes Plus Mechanisms

In one of the first modern textbooks in the field, MacMahon and Pugh describe the etiology of illness as a two-part sequence of events [127]. The first refers to causal events prior to the initial somatic response that marks the starting point of the disease process in an individual. The second consists of subsequent "mechanisms within the body leading from the initial response to the characteristic manifestations of the disease".[1]

In modern biomedicine, the first is frequently called *illness causation* and the second *pathomechanism*. The overarching story that explains illness occurrence, the *etiological stance* [21], unites causes and pathogenesis as the *causation process*, and pathogenesis plus clinical disease as the *disease process*. Note that we use the term *etiological process* to refer to the unity of both these overlapping processes (Fig. 3.1). Also, we use the terms *etiology* and *etiological process* synonymously.

In keeping with these notions, molecular epidemiologists describe the process that leads from causation to clinical disease as a four-stage sequence of intra-individual biological changes, including (i) internal dose, (ii) biologically effective dose, (iii) early biological effect, and (iv) altered structure/function [24]. In etiological terminology, this sequence describes the biological link between exposure (the cause) and onset of clinical disease. Using the same language, genomic epidemiologists Khoury and coauthors state that "disease is viewed as the result of a chain of events that comprise an intricate 'web' of external causal events and internal pathogenetic mechanisms" [150:12]. Thus, in a perfect world, interventions on causal events should help prevent illness. If risk factors were indeed causes, interventions on risk factors could be expected to do the same. This state of affairs is

[1] We see a direct line of thought here, coming from J.S. Mill (1806–1873) to J.L. Mackie (1917–81) to Ken Rothman. In the 1970's it was textbook knowledge that "just as any effect has multiple causes, the alteration of any cause may be expected to have multiple effects besides the one intended"; see [127], p.26. This view stands in stark contrast to the Henle-Koch postulates favored earlier; see [17], ch.2.

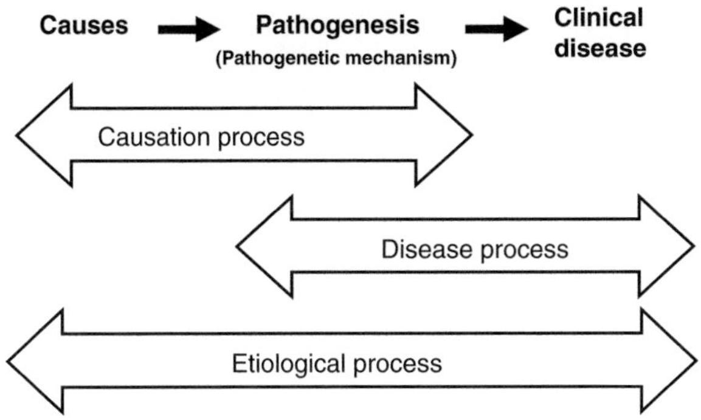

Fig. 3.1 Etiology conceptualized as a two-phase process. The causation process includes causes and the subsequent pathogenetic mechanism. The disease process includes the pathogenesis and clinical disease. Knowledge of the overarching etiological process can provide useful etiological explanations. (Reprinted with permission from Dammann [21])

accommodated by the sufficient-cause model described in next section, as well as both the dispositional and counterfactual accounts of causation addressed later in this chapter.

3.2.1 Hume and the Regularity Accounts of Causation

Perhaps Hume's greatest contribution to philosophy, and arguably the root of most philosophical discourse on the nature of causation, are his discussions of *necessary connexion* in his *Enquiry Concerning Human Understanding* and *A Treatise of Human Nature*. Hume argued that in order to have an *idea* of something, one must first have an *impression* of it. In other words, in order to understand a concept, and for it to be meaningful, one must first be able to directly observe it, e.g., we have a meaningful concept of *blue* only because we have directly observed blue objects (had an *impression* of blueness) and can now imagine (conjure up an *idea* of) the colour blue. If one had never seen the colour blue, it would be impossible to imagine the colour blue-indeed, the very concept of "blue" would be meaningless.

When we think about cause and effect, we have a tendency to think about one event producing, necessitating, or at a minimum increasing the probability of another. But what enables us to draw this inference? What do we see (that is, what do we have an *impression* of) in addition to "one event, followed by another" that gives meaning to the concept of n*ecessary connection*? Hume argues that the concept of necessary connection in the objects is entirely meaningless, since there is no directly observable necessitation relation.

Although he failed to recognise it at the time, Hume was the first to propose early forms of two distinct definitions of cause. The first has come to be known as the *regularity theory* and the second an embryonic form of the *counterfactual theory* of causation. We will discuss the latter, and its contribution to contemporary epidemiological methodology in Sect. 3.2.3. In this section we outline the origins of the regularity theory and its contribution to models of illness causation.

Hume initially defined a cause to be "an object, followed by another, and where all objects similar to the first are followed by objects similar to the second" [151:146]. In other words, *X* is a cause of *Y* if (i) events *X* and *Y* occur (ii) event *Y* occurs subsequent to event *X* (iii) whenever an event similar to event *X* occurs, an event similar to event *Y* occurs. He adds later that the two events must be spatially, as well as temporally contiguous (when the rock causes the window to smash, the rock must touch the window and do so right before the glass shatters). On the face of it, Hume's definition holds true of most causal events, e.g., when stung by a bee, swelling occurs. The swelling occurs shortly after the sting and every time we are stung by a bee, swelling occurs. So it is reasonable to conclude that the bee sting causes the swelling. On reflection, however, there are many counterexamples to this simple version of the regularity account. There are cases where an event of type A unquestionably causes an event of type B, and yet events of type A are not always followed by events of type B, e.g., unprotected sex may cause pregnancy, but it is not the case that every instance of unprotected sex is followed by pregnancy. Nevertheless, the basic regularity concept has been highly influential in medical discourse.

Many subsequent philosophers have accepted this link-like characterization of the relationship between two events deemed cause and effect; so many, in fact, that Chris Hitchcock entitled his critique of such metaphors *Of Humean Bondage*. He claims that defining causation as two facts bound by a causal relation makes little sense, because many characteristics of the different phenotypes of causation do not fit this rather rigid scheme. Hume's tendency to use metaphors of attachment in his discussions of causation, he argues, "has impeded progress in the philosophical study of causation". If "causes really were cemented to their effects … we would be able to develop tests for (its) presence" [152:3].

The Humean bond is probably also an accurate description of how most doctors, nurses, and patients think about illness causation, and it might even be the way some epidemiologists think about it. Above and beyond its convenient simplicity, it is probably also the illusion of testability (see Chap. 4) that makes this way of thinking about illness causation so attractive. However, the simplicity of *single cause attribution* [91] stands in sharp contrast to the multiple causation paradigm championed by the epidemiologist Kenneth Rothman, and the philosopher J.L. Mackie in the mid 1970s [33]. Their models are fundamentally a multifactorial form of Hume's regularity theory.[2]

[2] It remains to be shown whether non-linear dynamics analytic techniques, and other non-exact methods such as e.g., fuzzy logic [153], are superior to the currently available epidemiologic-statistical armamentarium.

3.2.2 *Rothman's Pies and Mackie's INUS Conditions*

In this section we discuss our first metaphysical conception of causation: the sufficient-component cause model, as summarized in the epidemiological literature by Ken Rothman in 1976 [33].

J.L. Mackie provides the first comprehensive discussion of this type of causal theory in his 1974 book *The Cement of the Universe*. He outlines a number of common causal scenarios that a plausible account of causation must accommodate, including cases of "overdetermination" (whereby more than one exposure is individually sufficient for the outcome, but none of them is necessary), and cases whereby several causal factors are individually insufficient, but together are sufficient for an outcome.

More formally, where *X* is an independent variable (the cause/exposure) and *Y* is a dependent variable (the effect/outcome):

1. *X* is necessary and sufficient for *Y*
   Both *X* and *Y* are always present together, and nothing but *X* is needed to cause *Y*. $x \rightarrow y$
2. *X* is necessary but not sufficient for *Y*.
   X must be present when *Y* is present, but *Y* is not always present when *X* is..., some additional factor must also be present. $x + z \rightarrow y$
3. *X* is not necessary but sufficient to cause *Y*.
   X may or may not be present when *Y* is present, because *Y* has other causes and can occur without *X*. For example, an enlarged spleen can have many separate causes that are unconnected with each other. $x \rightarrow y$; $w + z \rightarrow y$
4. *X* is neither necessary nor sufficient to cause *Y*.
   Again *X* may or may not be present when *Y* is present. Under these conditions, however, if *X* is present with *Y*, some additional factor must also be present. Here *X* is a contributory cause of *Y* in some causal sequences, $x + z \rightarrow y$; $w + z \rightarrow y$

When one takes the independent variables *X* to be a cause of disease, and the dependent variable *Y* to be disease occurrence (the start of the disease process), we see that this account of illness causation is inherently deterministic. To illustrate, consider Emma:

Emma is a young primary school teacher who in her first cold winter (CW) of teaching contracts the flu, which results in Emma being sick (ES). Two students in her class were sick with the same condition (take 1S to be *student 1 being sick*, 2S to be *student 2 being sick*), and it was they who exposed her to the virus. Emma opposes vaccination, so chose not to vaccinate herself against the flu virus that year (not-EV). In these circumstances (that is, *exposure to virus*; *cold weather*; and *no vaccination*), Emma determinately contracts flu. Were at least one of these conditions not met, Emma would (determinately) not contract flu. In the circumstances, the following statements are thus true:

1. Had Emma received the flu vaccination that year, she would not have contracted flu. (EV → not-ES)
2. Had the weather been warmer, Emma would not have contracted the flu. (not-CW → not-ES)
3. Had Emma not been exposed to the virus, she would not have contracted flu. (not-1S & not-2S → not-ES
4. Exposure to any one of the sick students is, in conjunction with the conditions of "cold weather", and "not vaccinated", sufficient for contracting the flu. ((1S & CW & not-EV) → ES) or (2S & CW & not-EV) → ES) or (1S & 2S & CW & not-EV) → ES))

From 4, note that given any of the three disjuncts in the antecedent, ES is determined. That is to say, Emma will contract flu with probability 1 so long as all conditions within any one of those three disjuncts are met.

To capture this model Mackie describes a *cause* as any *insufficient but non-redundant part of unnecessary by sufficient condition* (an INUS condition for short) for an effect (outcome). Rothman's sufficient-cause model is in essence a notational variant of Mackie's. In Rothman's model, each *piece* of his causal pies (Fig. 3.2) translates as a unique INUS condition, and only when a pie is complete (all the pieces for at least one pie are in place) will the outcome manifest. Of course, the sufficient-component cause model is not primarily designed for *singular causation* (such as Emma's flu). Typically, epidemiologists are more interested in general causal claims; that is, what exposures caused disease *D*, as opposed what exposure caused a particular instance of *D*. But this is well-accommodated by the sufficient-component cause model, since each pie represents a unique way of contracting a disease.

Figure 3.3 shows the pies representing the sufficient causes for Emma contracting the flu, as described above. Note that we have included a fourth piece, "all other causally relevant factors", since there are many non-redundant causal factors for Emma's contracting the flu not captured by the three conditions highlighted above e.g., *presence of lungs*, and *not wearing a biohazard suit*. These conditions must be

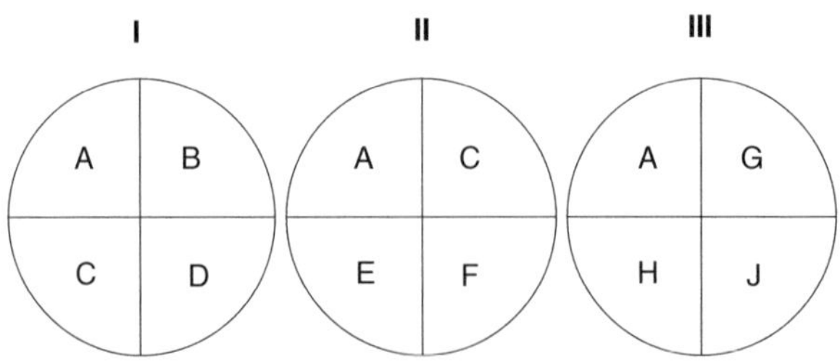

Fig. 3.2 Rothman's pies I – III depict three complete constellations of causes that, together, are sufficient to result in illness occurrence. Each piece of the pies A – J represents a component cause that is in itself insufficient to cause the illness. Only one of the component causes, A, is necessary for illness causation by virtue of being the one component to complete all three possible pies

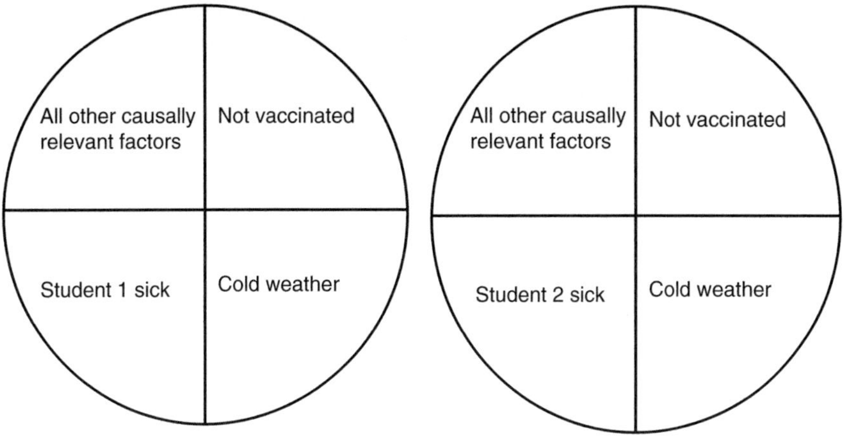

Fig. 3.3 Sufficient causes for Emma's flu

considered a part of each sufficient cause, but given that they are often considered uninformative/irrelevant, it is easier to group them together into a single piece.[3]

Some have argued that the INUS condition/causal pie model is problematic. Objections include: who might be the pies' cook [41]; that is to say, who chooses which pieces make up the pie?; and the fact that this model fails to include temporal aspects of disease causation. The first problem, we argue, is not an issue for the sufficient-cause model. From a metaphysical perspective, there are a plurality of possible states of affairs that can lead to Emma getting the flu - there are many pies. We do not get to choose what the pies are, since the content of the pies is ultimately governed by natural organizing principles [154]. What we can do is choose which pieces to group together and label 'other causal factors', and which to pick out as more salient (most commonly those subject to interventions).

It is clear that both Mackie and Rothman endorse a multifactorial and non-selective approach to illness causation; but Rothman points out that although each piece of the pie is, strictly speaking, as much a cause as any other, some pieces have greater explanatory value than others. It is those with the greatest explanatory value that clinicians and population health interventionists are interested in, and thus it is those that should be picked out from all the other causally relevant factors. Of course, we are often bad at choosing which causal factors are salient and which are not, and we are often unaware of some (or all) of the complex causal states of affairs that will lead to the onset of a particular disease - but this is a problem for medicine and public health, not for the model of illness causation. In this way, the sufficient-component cause model can easily overcome the *who cooks the pie* objection.

[3] We have come to call this concept *combined contribution*; see [21].

Arguably, the second objection is more problematic. The induction time of some causal factors is longer than that of others. Often genetic predispositions are causally relevant and present since conception. The event that triggers the disease associated with this predisposition, on the other hand, will be simultaneous with, or at least not too long before the onset of the start of the disease process. Rothman recognises this when he states that "cancer itself has often been characterised as a disease process with a long induction-time, but this characterisation is a misconception. Any late-acting component in the causal process… will have a short induction time, and the induction time will always be zero for the last component cause… because after the last component cause acts, disease has occurred" [155:29]. By considering each component piece as distinct, the sufficient-component cause model *prima facie* permits one to attribute different induction times to each causally relevant component. However, the complete pie does not in fact contain this information, since the induction time of a component piece is not relevant to the completion of the sufficient cause.

It may be true that sufficient-cause models (Rothman and Mackie) cannot contain information concerning the induction time of their component pieces, but to some extent this is a straw man, since knowing the component pieces alone is sufficient to enable epidemiologists to search for suitable interventions. Epidemiologists may need to independently investigate the nature of the component pieces, and this process may include discovering induction times, but the full causal story from the moment the patient moves from a state of health to a state of disease is already captured by the sufficient-cause models produced by Rothman and Mackie.

Rothman's pies provide a model of illness causation according to which the relata of the causal relation are (i) those causal factors that together initiate the onset of disease, and (ii) the beginning of the disease course. However, we have not yet discussed the pathogenetic mechanisms – those biological processes that lead from the moment of causation to the onset of a disease. This etiological second step comprises a sequence of pathophysiological processes within an organism's body, which is not explicitly captured by sufficient-cause models.

We do not take this to be a significant flaw. The sufficient-cause(s) of any specific physiological state can, in principle, be modelled using Rothman's method, and thus effective interventions might be identified even after the onset of disease. However, other metaphysical accounts of causation, in addition to providing a model of illness causation, paint a picture of the *nature* of disease, by paying more attention to the nature of the causal processes leading from the beginning of the disease course, through to its completion (death or cure). In Sect. 3.2.4 we outline the increasingly popular "dispositional account" of causation, and how recently, some philosophers of medicine [156, 157] take this to best capture the nature of disease.

3.2.3 The Counterfactual Account of Causation

Alongside his regularity theory of causation, Hume writes that one can identify a cause wherever "if the first object had not been, the second never existed" [151:146]. This idea is mirrored by philosopher David Lewis, who states "if *c* and *e* are two actual events such that *e* would not have occurred without *c*, then *c* is a cause of *e*." [9:563], and in the numerous "difference-making" definitions of cause, e.g., the *pragmatic* definition given by Mervyn Susser, which holds simply that "a cause is what makes a difference" [38].

To illustrate, take A and B to be two distinct events: Sam having unprotected sexual intercourse with Jo (who is HIV positive) (*A*), and Sam later being diagnosed as HIV positive (*B*).[4] The 'counterfactual' analysis of causation provides a methodology for determining whether a causal relation stands between A and B. It states that "if *A* caused *B*, then both *A* and *B* occurred, and (in the circumstances) if *A* had not occurred then *B* would not have occurred… (where *A* and *B* are logically and conceptually distinct events)"[10:37]. Sam having sexual intercourse with Jo caused Sam's positive HIV test only if (i) Sam and Jo had sex, *and* (ii) if Sam had not had sex with Jo, Sam would not be HIV positive. Having sex with Jo made a difference.[5]

Although it is beyond the scope of this book to delve deeply into the metaphysics of counterfactual theories of causation, the most prominent views in the contemporary philosophy literature are based on Lewis's possible world semantics. The idea, crudely speaking, is that to determine whether event *A* causes event *B*, one looks at a possible world in which all states of affairs are identical except for the fact that *A* does not occur. If, in that possible world, *B* does not occur, then event *A* is a cause of event *B* in the actual world.[6] One might object that this admits of far too many causes in the medical context and indeed this view, like Mackie's, is non-selective. That is to say, the presence of oxygen in the room is as much a cause of Emma getting the flu as her lack of immunity to the virus and her students being sick. However, as Rothman argued, accepting that the presence of oxygen is a cause does not prevent us from attributing different explanatory weights to different causes. We can and do select the most salient causal factors for the purposes of clinical medicine.

Although the philosophical account presented above is (unlike the sufficient-cause model) very much targeted at singular causation, this approach has inspired some of the most influential methodologies in modern epidemiology. These include the *potential outcomes approach* (POA), which is sometimes even referred to as *the counterfactual approach*), as well as the form of clinical study commonly deemed the gold standard, the randomised controlled trial (RCT).

An RCT employs one of a number of randomisation strategies to ensure that any difference between the exposure group and the contrast groups can be attributed to the exposure; the assumption being that if those members of the exposure group had not received the treatment under investigation, the outcomes would have been iden-

[4] A and B are distinct, not in the sense that they are causally unrelated, but insofar as the event 'having sexual intercourse' and the event 'being diagnosed HIV positive' are spatiotemporally non-identical.

[5] *Making a difference* does mean *causing* the difference. Merely being associated with a difference would not make a difference.

[6] This simplified version is problematic in cases of overdetermination such as that described with our primary school teacher Emma, since even if student 1 had not been sick, Emma would still have contracted the flu, since student 2 being sick was sufficient. The more nuanced versions of Lewis's metaphysic avoid these issues, however.

tical to those of the control group. Of course, to more closely adhere to the principles of Hume and Lewis, the exposure group and control group would have to comprise the exact same members at the exact same time, and for obvious reasons this is impossible. Nevertheless, RCTs are designed precisely to demonstrate the difference a specified exposure makes to a population.

The POA operates on a similar premise [130]. Unlike the metaphysical account of causation as counterfactual dependence, it focuses on measuring the effect of one intervention *versus* another. The POA is thus a tool for measuring the relative causal effects of practicable interventions.

What is unique about the POA is that the effect size of one exposure is measured relative to the effect of some other, contrary-to-fact (and thus unobservable) exposure. A POA study requires just one actual intervention, *x1*, where O is a measure of outcome and O(*x1*) is the outcome among individuals with exposure *x1*. Since *x1* is the only actual intervention, the measurements O(*xn*) for all values of *n* other than *1* are contrary-to-fact – they are the *potential outcomes*. In order to measure the causal effect of the actual exposure *x1* one compares O(*x1*) with the outcome of some contrary-to-fact exposure *xc*. In this way, one can (by estimating the potential outcome O(*x0*)) measure the causal effect of intervention *x1* versus *x0* e.g., if *x1* is *immunised against the flu* and *x0* is *not immunised against the flu*, one can estimate the risk of contracting the flu due to not being immunised versus being immunised by O(*x0*)/O(*x1*). This comparative methodology makes statements such as *eating red meat causes bowel cancer* meaningless by themselves; there must be a potential outcome against which it is measured, e.g., compared to vegetarianism, *eating red meat increases risk of bowel cancer.*

As one of us has argued elsewhere [156], we reiterate here that the link between the Humean/Lewisian accounts of causation as counterfactual dependence, and the POA, is tenuous for at least two reasons. First, the philosophical account is an analysis of singular causation. That is to say, it is about token events causing other token events. Both RCTs and the outcomes of POA studies make general causal claims - whereas Lewis wants to know whether smoking caused Leslie's cancer, RCTs and the POA try to establish whether smoking causes cancer (versus not smoking). Second, Hume and Lewis are trying to put together a metaphysical account of what causation *is*. Epidemiologists have the more pragmatic goal of discovering what the effect of an exposure is. That said it is clear that the philosophical account of causation as counterfactual dependence – of something/some event that makes a difference – has had a profound effect on epidemiologic methodology.

3.2.4 Dispositions: The Powers of Disease

Thus far we have discussed the regularity (the set of analyses under which the sufficient-cause model falls) and counterfactual theories of causation in the context of illness causation. More recently, however, both illness causation and pathogenesis have been looked at through the lens of a third metaphysic: dispositionalism [156–158].

Some dispositionalists, such as Alexander Bird, prefer to restrict this metaphysic to fundamental properties, that is to say, only the fundamental properties such as charge and mass have a dispositional nature. Others [98, 156, 157] are, at least on a conceptual level, happy to extend dispositionalism to all causal interactions,[7] at both the microscopic and macroscopic levels.

Dispositionalism is the theory that at least some properties have a *dispositional* nature, and that these properties are (at least in part) responsible for how objects behave (including all physiological systems and pathogens). The property *mass* is dispositional since it confers a range of dispositions on the objects instantiating it, e.g., to accelerate at rate directly proportional to the force applied to it. The mass of an object does not *necessitate* its acceleration towards another massive object, however. There may be some external force preventing this movement (perhaps a third object with mass pulling it in the opposite direction). The dispositionalist metaphysic, then, permits an object to have the disposition to behave in manner *E* under conditions *C*, but may nevertheless fail to do so even when *C* is met.

Objects instantiate many dispositional properties; some are fundamental (such as mass), but those who grant macroscopic dispositions claim that many *emerge* from the more fundamental properties. A vase is *fragile* (the disposition) and disposed to smash (the manifestation) when it hits the ground. Of course, *fragility* is not a fundamental property - a vase's fragility emerges from the fundamental properties instantiated by its parts, and the arrangement of those parts – but it is a dispositional property nonetheless. In this way, human beings and other organisms are disposed to develop disease under certain conditions. A causal interaction involves the manifestation of dispositions of *all* objects involved in that interaction. The malaria virus is disposed to make human beings sick, but if the agent exposed to the virus has taken prophylactics her disposition to contract the disease is diminished. In other words, when consumed, the dispositions of the medication affect the dispositions of the agent, such that the disposition of the virus to make humans sick is attenuated.

Illness causation and intervention becomes *a battle of the dispositions*, since all human beings (to a lesser or greater extent) are disposed to get diseases under certain conditions. In the case of infectious diseases, our immune systems play a large role. One's immune system is significantly weakened following chemotherapy, and thus one's disposition to contract infectious diseases substantially increases. Dietary factors, HIV, and many genetic factors all contribute in similar ways. It's not just infectious diseases, of course. All human beings (and many other animals), for example, are disposed to have seizures under certain conditions (excessive stress, lack of sleep, drug withdrawal, and so on). Diagnosed epileptics are typically more disposed towards seizures than patients healthy in that regard, of course, but nevertheless we all have the disposition.

When the etiological process of an infectious disease begins, the dispositions the patient has (in virtue of white blood cells etc) to fight off infection fail. It is not just

[7] If not explicitly indicated, causal *interaction* does not refer to statistical interaction between causes, but to whatever interaction needs to be present to render a cause-effect relationship causal.

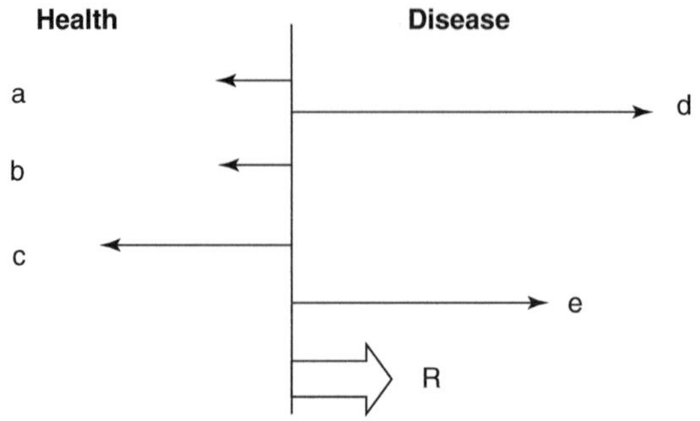

Fig. 3.4 The Mumford-Anjum Model: characteristics as dispositions away from (a, b, c) or towards health (d, e). The relative strength of these dispositions in turn disposes towards recovery (R). (Reprinted with permission from Smart, Concepts and causes in the philosophy of disease, Palgrave, 2017, p. 58)

the dispositions of the virus that manifest, however; the dispositions of the patient to become infected also play a role (a table won't become infected, since tables do not have the requisite dispositions). Illness causation thus requires the "mutual manifestation" of both the dispositions of the pathogen and the patient.

A good way of modelling this was presented by Mumford and Anjum [98] and later adapted to medicine by Smart [156] and Fuller [157].

Following Mumford and Anjum, the *vector* model of causation depicted in Fig. 3.4 represents five distinct dispositions: *a, b* and *c* dispose the patient not to contract an infectious disease, to varying degrees. Take *a* to be the agent's distance from the viral exposure, *b* to be her wearing of a surgical mask, and *c* to be her ideal white blood cell count. These all dispose the agent *away* from contracting the disease, with the ideal white blood cell count playing a bigger role than the surgical mask as indicated by the size of the vector. Vectors *d* and *e*, on the other hand, dispose the agent *towards* contracting the disease. Take *d* to be the virus's high degree of pathogenicity, and *e* to be the length of time exposed to the virus. R is the resultant vector. In this case it tells us that, overall, the agent tends towards contracting the disease – the longer the resultant vector, the more likely she is to get sick. Using this model, clinicians can provide interventions in many different ways e.g., use disinfectants to kill bacteria before coming into contact with patients; improve patients' immune systems by administering vaccinations; using antibiotics to cure infections before more serious conditions develop, and so on.

Pathogenesis and Ontology (or What Is a Disease?)

One of us has argued elsewhere that diseases are processes of mutually manifesting causal dispositions [159]. More recently, Fuller has argued that chronic diseases are not the processes themselves, but the dispositions of patients that give rise to those processes [157]. In the case of epilepsy, for example, Fuller argues that the disease comprises the patient's (more potent than is normal) disposition to have seizures. We agree with Fuller that at least some chronic diseases have this character. It is not the case that epileptics are in a constant state of seizure, and the frequency of seizures can often be reduced or even eliminated with the appropriate medication. An epileptic does not cease to have the condition as soon as a seizure ends, and someone without epilepsy can have a one-off seizure - it is the abnormally strong disposition to have seizures that makes one epileptic. It is thus worth distinguishing between *diseases* and *dise*ase-processes, or a *disease-course*.

Fuller does not intend to provide a metaphysic of disease that generalises across all diseases. He "focus[es] on the nature of chronic diseases rather than all diseases, sacrificing generality for sound induction. The class of all diseases is heterogeneous. We might expect greater metaphysical diversity within it, which would limit the generalizations we can make about diseases" [157:3202]. Again, we find ourselves in agreement. Whereas the concept of a disease as a "disposition to E" seems to fit well with chronic diseases such as epilepsy, this is not the case for infectious diseases.

It is perfectly normal to be disposed to contract highly contagious diseases in the *right* circumstances. One might argue that someone without this disposition (via immunity or some other protective characteristic) is healthier than [160] someone with it, but being disposed towards contracting bubonic plague is certainly not sufficient for having the condition, or indeed being unhealthy more generally. In the case of infectious diseases, a metaphysic of diseases as "causal processes best seen as simultaneously acting sequences of mutually manifesting dispositions"[159:252] that lead up to and include undesirable symptoms/subnormal physiological part-function, seems more appropriate than the patient's prior disposition to contract the infection.

3.3 Summary

In this chapter we have discussed two linked but essentially distinct issues concerning causation in medicine and population health. First we considered numerous ways in which the concept of a cause in illness causation can be cashed out, and second, we examined a causal interpretation of the *nature* of illness; that is to say, what a disease *is* from a metaphysical perspective. Although there are numerous other ways in which the latter task has been approached e.g., the disease entity model [161], at least one plausible interpretation of the nature of disease is grounded by an account of causation now well established in philosophical discourse.

Having established the distinction between a number of stages in the etiological process (whereby *illness causation* concerns the causes/causal chains of events leading up to the onset of the initial somatic response that marks the start of the disease process, *pathogenesis* concerns the causes/causal processes leading from the initial response to those symptoms characteristic of the disease, the term *causal process* (in this context) combines illness causation with pathogenesis, *disease process* unites pathogenesis with clinical disease, and the *etiological process* unites all of the above, from illness causation to clinical disease) we discussed four conceptual analyses of cause, namely the Humean "regularity" approach, Rothman and Mackie's sufficient cause/*INUS* condition model, Lewis's counterfactual account, and the dispositional conceptual analysis of causation defended by Mumford and Anjum (amongst others). Each philosophical analysis is mirrored in medical practice and epidemiological research, some more accurately and with better consequences than others.

Hume's basic regularity theory takes an event *a* to be a cause of event *b* where all events of type A (those events qualitatively similar to event *a*) are followed by events of type B. It is ultimately an account of general causation that informs one of causal relations between particular events via general causal claims such as A's cause B's. This view is *prima facie* plausible, since the application of general causal claims is frequently linked to singular cases – the patient's heart failure caused her death since heart failure causes death – but it faces a plethora of counterexamples and other conceptual issues (not least the fact that most of the time, exceptionless regularities in medicine, as elsewhere, are very rare indeed). This is troublesome, since it seems to be the way many doctors, nurses, patients (and to some extent even epidemiologists) seem to view illness causation.

Following Mackie, Rothman's sufficient-component cause model implicitly takes individual causes to be "insufficient but non-redundant parts of unnecessary but sufficient conditions". This view is compelling insofar as it accommodates the intuition that a plausible model of illness causation should be multifactorial. It is, in fact, a more sophisticated form of the regularity account of causation, insofar as when *all* of the pie's pieces are replicated, the same outcome is inevitable. However, its more sophisticated, multifactorial nature eliminates many of the problems that render Hume's account implausible. As a regularity account it is also one that provides general causal claims, but generally only about multiple causes when united. It is thus more accommodating of exceptions and permits causal claims such as *smoking causes cancer* despite the fact that many smokers never get cancer.

In this chapter we outlined the counterfactual account in two distinct ways. The first was the non-discriminatory view of singular causation proposed by Lewis in terms of possible world semantics (and previously by Hume), and the second, supposedly inspired by those philosophical views, the POA - an account of general causation commonly employed by contemporary epidemiologists. The differences between the two analyses of causation are substantial, but they share one common factor: that only one potential outcome is actual. The causal influence of the intervention under investigation is determined by comparing the effects of intervention to counterfactual (non-actualised) situations (no intervention, or different interventions). In the medical context, this implies the causal effect is determined by comparing the outcome of a study on intervention, with the assumed outcome of a study that never takes place. This method has clear limitations, some of which we discuss in the next chapter, but it admits of estimating causal effects that would otherwise be impossible to quantify.

The final metaphysical/conceptual account of causation we discussed was the dispositional account, according to which patients are disposed towards becoming ill, and certain states of affairs dispose towards disease. Causation occurs when an effect occurs in virtue of the mutual manifestation of the dispositions of the patient and the dispositions of those disease-causing states of affairs, in the form of a disease process. This admits of both singular and general causal claims, although the general causal claims do not take the form of regularities, but *tendencies*. The dispositional account is useful from a health care perspective, since it seems to more accurately model the nature of the etiological process, and importantly, the nature of interventions. It also provides interesting insights into the nature of diseases themselves. Indeed, as Fuller observes, chronic diseases just seem to *be* certain (undesirable) dispositions that patients with those diseases instantiate.

The concepts of causation employed in the health sciences are integral to their practice, whether used consciously or unconsciously. It should be apparent, then, that a clear insight into the nature of the metaphysical and conceptual schemes underlying the etiological process would help all those working in medicine and population health.

Chapter 4
Causal Inference in Population Health Informatics

Abstract Having discussed the metaphysics of disease etiology in Chap. 3, in this chapter we discuss a number of important epistemological problems concerning causal inference in medicine and population health informatics. With origins tracing back to at least the eighteenth century, the problem of induction (that is, the problem of justifying inferences from observed data to likely future or unobserved outcomes) is one of the most discussed issues in the philosophical literature. Given that causal inference plays such a large role in the health sciences and that all causal inferences are inductive in kind, we take a detailed look at how those working in the health sciences go about identifying, and justifying their causal claims. With this in mind, we examine Austin Bradford Hill's heuristics for causal inference in epidemiology, and argue that the postulation of criteria such as Hill's is nothing but a replacement of one dilemma with another: why should it be easier to identify the truth condition of the heuristics, than identifying the truth condition of the relationship between exposure and effect if they were hard and fast criteria? We conclude by asking whether genuine medical knowledge is possible. We outline a number of historically popular responses to the ultimate question in epistemology: "what is knowledge", and demonstrate the profound effect one's answer to that question has on the ability to claim medical knowledge of any form.

Keywords Epistemology of medicine · Causal inference · Hill's criteria · Problem of induction · Philosophy of epidemiology · Philosophy of public health

4.1 Introduction

In the previous chapter we examined the metaphysics of causation in population health. We considered a number of conceptual analyses of "cause", alongside the ontological commitments that accompany those accounts. We explained how these different approaches to causation affect the manner in which different aspects of disease etiology are viewed in the medical sciences and outlined how some concepts of cause are more useful than others depending on the circumstances in which they are used. In this chapter, we deal with a related (but distinct) issue in population health informatics: the problem of causal inference. This is an epistemological issue

O. Dammann, B. Smart, *Causation in Population Health Informatics and Data Science*, https://doi.org/10.1007/978-3-319-96307-5_4

as opposed to a metaphysical one; that is to say, this chapter concerns whether, when, and how can we accurately identify causal relationships between exposures and the onset of disease. An understanding of the nature of causation and insights into causal inference in the health sciences are intrinsically linked, of course, since it is through our understanding of the nature of causation that our causal inferences are made. Here we discuss the nature of this relationship, and analyze a number of ways in which epidemiologists and clinicians draw causal conclusions. Much of our discussion in this chapter and indeed in this book comes from work in philosophy of medicine. Still, it will become obvious why and how these discussion points are also relevant for causal inference in public/population health. We conclude by asking the question: "is genuine medical knowledge even possible?"

Medical researchers use a variety of experimental and statistical techniques to identify causal relationships. One might plausibly argue, in fact, that the core goal of medical research is to identify and quantify causation, whether it be in the identification of causes of disease, or in identifying effective interventions. The literature leaves us puzzled with regard to the following apparent disconnect, however: on the one hand, those working in the medical sciences frequently do not have much more than a vague definition of what a cause is in biomedicine and the life sciences (and even once more robust definitions of "cause" are applied, philosophical analysis of strategies in epidemiology highlight difficulties in justifying causal conclusions). On the other hand, researchers and clinicians are often rather happy with the results of our actions based on that vague understanding. In particular, we act as if we *know* how to identify causation, i.e., we act as if we truly know how to make correct causal inferences from observed data.

Although folk concepts of causality acquired by everybody on a daily basis may help someone learn that flipping a light switch is a great strategy if the goal is to illuminate the room at night, it misses most of the causal complexity in biomedicine in (a) different levels of causal sub-process (molecular, cell-cell, organ, person) and (b) qualitatively different ways how causes contribute to outcomes. The deeper understanding of causal concepts and the metaphysics of causation discussed in the previous chapter, in addition to a number of other philosophical issues to be introduced in this chapter, will help us assess the reliability of modern strategies for identifying causal relationships in medicine.

4.2 Causal Judgements

4.2.1 Three Fundamental Problems

Following on from those conclusions drawn by David Hume, cancer epidemiologist and theoretician of illness causation Douglas Weed writes, in the context of illness causation, that.

> causation cannot be seen. Causation cannot be proven … Nor can causation be made certain. It is, at best, an expert's judgment, at worst, an expert's guess. [61]

In a footnote, however, Weed adds that "it is reasonable to assume that some scientists' judgments are better than others" [61]. How can that be, however, if any judgment about causation would need to be judged against a solid reference frame? Weed offers a concise summary of three fundamental causal problems that, taken together, explain why causal hypotheses can never be true (see [61], footnote 14).

First, the *fundamental problem of causal inference*: we cannot observe in the same individual both the effect of an intervention and the non-effect in its absence. Weed's fundamental problem stems from the counterfactual account of causation discussed in Chap. 3 – that event *c* causes event *e* if and only if, if *c* had not occurred then *e* would not have occurred. If at a specific time *t*, event *c* occurs, we can observe what happens in that immediate vicinity afterwards; but we cannot observe at *t* what would have occurred if *c* had not occurred, since that state of affairs never materialised. Epidemiologists try to accommodate these problems through randomization and 'potential outcome' strategies, but to what extent these are successful is questionable. (We will return to this in Sect. 4.4.1.)

Second, the *fundamental problem of causal logic*: scientific evidence can never determine whether the causal hypothesis, alternative hypotheses, or chance determined the particular situation.

Third, that problem first identified by David Hume, *the fundamental problem of causation*: that causation is not observable - we see only the evidence, not causation itself. The fundamental problem of causation inevitably leads to the problem of induction (the focus of Sect. 4.3).

We thus have to think about ways how to proactively manage such risks. We do not want to accept illness, resulting from diseases, disorders, and accidents and their consequences as something given, inevitable, and unchangeable. We have agreed on effective ways to do something. This is the interventionist stance of medicine and public health. While medicine is devoted to post-hoc attempts to reduce suffering after the fact by treating illness pharmacologically, psychologically, or surgically, public health focuses on pre-hoc interventions designed to reduce the effects of health hazards via prevention. These aims have at least one thing in common, though: causal knowledge.

4.2.2 Explanation and Medical Knowledge

The debate about whether *evidence based medicine* (EBM) or *patient centred medicine* should take centre stage in contemporary clinical practice is ongoing. Practitioners of EBM hold that the evidence provided by epidemiological studies provides better justification for clinical decisions than expert opinion based on experience, intuition, and even pathological reasoning. They hold that whether an individual should be treated (and how) depends first on the results of clinical trials [133]. This, they argue, limits the risk of prescribing inefficient and/or harmful treatments. EBM contrasts with patient centred care, which prioritises the values and needs of the patient. Whereas the main concern of evidence based medicine is disease (the causes of disease and post-hoc and pre-hoc interventions), patient-centred care has "a humanistic, biopsychosocial perspective, combining ethical values on the 'ideal physician', with psychotherapeutic theories on facilitating patients' disclosure of real worries, and negotiation theories on decision making" [162:17].

Although patient centred care prioritises the values and needs of the patient, just as evidence based practitioners cannot ignore the needs of the patient, so those proponents of patient centred care must make clinical decisions in part based on the evidence from clinical trials. The way doctors think and act is thus, across the board, rooted in the concept of evidence. We will refer to evidence-based public health in Sect. 7.1.1.

Following the popularity of EBM, the biomedical community has developed ways to diagnose, treat, and predict outcomes based primarily on evidence from clinical trials over personal experience. Biomedical evidence mainly comprises empirical data supporting those inferences integral to clinical decision making, which in turn (we hope) leads to "knowledge" in medicine. As we shall discuss in greater depth in Sect. 4.7, the starting point of any philosopher's education in epistemology is Plato's definition of knowledge as "justified true belief" (JTB) [163]. Despite the problems with the JTB account, most attempts to capture the concept of knowledge include some form of "justification" criterion. Ideally, evidence in the form of biomedical data provides the justification for our beliefs, and perhaps they even contribute to their being true.

4.3 Knowledge

4.3.1 The Problem of Induction

In Chap. 3 we outlined Hume's "regularity" theory of causation, according to which event *c* causes event *e* if and only if:

1. Events of type *c* and events of type *e* are constantly conjoined i.e., an event of type *c* is always followed by an event of type *e*.
2. Event *c* is temporally prior to event *e*.
3. There is contiguity i.e., the objects involved in the causal process physically touch one another in some way.
4. There is a necessary connection between those events, but where the idea of "necessary connection" is copied from a feeling of inevitability, rather than an observation of anything in the world (since there is nothing "in the objects" to observe over and above one event followed by another). Necessary connection, for Hume, is in the mind, not in the objects.

Whether or not one accepts the regularity theory of causation (and we have reason to think that medical and public health professionals in some contexts do (see Chap. 3)), the empiricist attitudes leading to Hume's conclusions highlight a problem in justifying causal inferences in population health. If one cannot observe necessary connection in the objects, it is not clear that events of one type *have* to follow the events identified as their causes (or even whether the probability of the effect is increased by its cause).

Let us continue with Hume to generalise the problem. In *The Enquiry Concerning Human Understanding* Hume identifies two kinds of proposition. He calls these *relations of ideas* and *matters of fact*. The former concern only concepts and tell us nothing about the nature of the world. *All bachelors are unmarried men* is a proposition of this kind; it is analytically true, since to be a bachelor just *is* to be an unmarried man. *Matters of fact*, on the other hand, are propositions that provide information about the world around us. "Carbon emissions contribute to climate change" tells us something about climate change that is not contained within the concept of *climate change*. This proposition provides causal information, but there are many *matters of fact* that do not: "The Suez Canal passes through Egypt" is not a *relation of ideas* because its content is not confined to concepts, but rather provides information about the world. The medical knowledge we are concerned with in this chapter exclusively concerns matters of fact.

We know with certainty that, tomorrow, all bachelors will be unmarried men – it is in the meaning of the concept. But do I know that "if I consume plenty of cyanide tomorrow then I will suffer"? One might claim to be certain of it, but consider on what grounds one is so certain. We believe that cyanide harms humans because every time a human being has consumed cyanide, he/she has been harmed. Given our knowledge of past events, it seems rational to believe that cyanide is always pathologic, so it is rational to believe that consuming cyanide tomorrow will cause harm. This causal inference corresponds perfectly with Hume's regularity theory of causation: there is contiguity, constant conjunction, temporal priority, and necessary connection (in the mind). But with nothing observable over and above those 4 criteria – with no necessary connection *in the objects* - there is no *prima facie* justification for drawing conclusions about future instances of cyanide consumption.

This problem, commonly known as *the problem of induction*, generalises to all inductive inferences – how can one justify any predictions [or inferences from particular instances to generalisations (e.g. "all *observed* cases of gangrene require treatment" to "*all* cases of gangrene require treatment")] based on past observations? If we take the problem of induction seriously, it is a problem for clinicians and epidemiologists alike, since all studies, prognoses, and treatment programs rely heavily on inductive reasoning. If we cannot use past observations to make predictions or generalisations, all clinical trials become redundant. If no causal inferences are justified, we cannot predict a disease course, and we cannot predict which interventions will be effective. Induction is the very cornerstone of medical reasoning.[1]

It is tempting not to be concerned about the problem of induction. After all, we rely on induction constantly (we don't put our hands in boiling water, since experience of one form or another tells us that's unwise!), and it is generally a highly

[1] The alternative would be to acknowledge *medical nihilism* as discussed by Jacob Stegenga [164].

successful strategy – but the problem should not be taken lightly, particularly in the sciences. We only have to look at the history of medicine to see why.

In Ancient Greece the theory of humorism was widely adopted. Hippocates (c. 460 BC – c. 370 BC), a man often viewed as the father of modern medicine and a figure still highly influential in medical ethics (in particular through the *Hippocratic Oath* [165]), is attributed with the following description of illness causation:

> The Human body contains blood, phlegm, yellow bile and black bile. These are the things that make up its constitution and cause its pains and health. Health is primarily that state in which these constituent substances are in the correct proportion to each other, both in strength and quantity, and are well mixed. Pain occurs when one of the substances presents either a deficiency or an excess, or is separated in the body and not mixed with others. [166:262]

The humoral theory enjoyed popularity for over 2000 years, so its demise may have been surprising to many, but even if interventions based on that theory had at times been successful, there was no logical contradiction when the theory was falsified.

One might also be tempted to think that since the humoral theories were replaced by germ theory, and antibiotics, antiseptics and effective anaesthesia became commonplace, medicine has progressed to the extent that we no longer need to worry about our inductions being unjustified. But even now, accepted theories based on empirical studies are regularly refuted. Take the following example concerning child nutrition.

A project funded by The World Bank set out to improve child malnutrition rates in Tamil Nadu State, India. Food supplements and additional health measures were provided, and mothers of malnourished children were educated in nutrition. As a result, malnutrition rates in the area dropped significantly. The success of the project motivated the inductive move from "food supplements and educating mothers reduces child malnutrition in Tamil Nadu", to the general hypothesis that "food supplements and educating mothers reduces child malnutrition". The World Bank's project was subsequently extended to Bangladesh, where there is a similar problem. The very same measures were put in place, but this time there was no drop in child malnutrition whatsoever. Two explanations for the discrepancy were proposed: first, that "food supplied by the project was used not as a supplement but as a substitute, with the usual food allocation for that child passing to another member of the family" [167:983], and second that "the program targeted the mothers of young children. But [in Bangladesh] mothers are frequently not the decision makers… with respect to health and nutrition of their children" (White, 2009 as cited in [167:984]). These background conditions were not taken into consideration when the initial inductive extrapolations from Tamil Nadu to Bangladesh were made, but they couldn't have been, since these conditions were, at the time, unknown. In medicine, and in the sciences more generally, this is regularly the case. There can be unknown confounders, there can be interfering factors present elsewhere that were not present in observed instances, and so on. It is unsurprising, then, that inductive inferences are fragile, even within the current medical paradigm.

John Ioannidis explains in his 2005 paper that:

> Published research findings are sometimes refuted by subsequent evidence, with ensuing confusion and disappointment. Refutation and controversy is seen across the range of research designs, from clinical trials and traditional epidemiological studies to the most modern molecular research. There is increasing concern that in modern research, false findings may be the majority or even the vast majority of published research claims. However, this should not be surprising. It can be proven that most claimed research findings are false. [168]

A number of reasons for the prevalence of false positives in clinical trials have been put forward, including implicit biases and pressure from those funding the research, but ultimately all medical knowledge falls out of evidence gathered through experience, and is thus subject to the problem of induction. So to what extent is medical knowledge justified? If inductive reasoning is universally unjustified, little or perhaps even no medical knowledge is justified. And given that justification is generally considered a precondition for knowledge, medical knowledge could be far more scarce than one might think. We shall return to the question of whether medical knowledge exists in Sect. 4.7.

4.3.2 *Solutions to the Problem of Induction*

4.3.2.1 The Inductive Solution

Despite the many scientific theories that have ultimately been refuted, it is probably fair to say that most *every day hypotheses* based on inductive reasoning enjoy continued success. We expect to stick to the ground every morning (due to past experiences of gravity), and thus far there have been no exceptions; we expected the sun to rise yesterday, and it did; we expected those antibiotics to fight off the infection, and the infection went away. As a result, one obvious solution to the problem is that although induction is fallible, it has been largely successful in the past, so we should expect it to continue to be successful.

The problem with this solution is obvious. To reason from the past success of induction to the future success of induction is itself an inductive inference. We are using induction to justify induction, so the argument is circular.

4.3.2.2 Inference to the Best Explanation

Inerence to the best explanation" (also known as *abduction*) is a principle that states that one should believe the hypothesis that best explains some phenomenon. This argument is often used by scientific realists, who claim that one should believe the entities postulated by scientific theories to exist as scientists describe them (such as electrons in electron theory), since the existence of those entities best explain why the predictions based on those theories are successful. It is the explanatory power of the theory that justifies one's belief that it is true. Whether or not one wishes to be a scientific realist, inference to the best explanation is appealing. The best explanation for smokers getting lung cancer more frequently than non-smokers is that smoking causes cancer, so we should believe that smoking causes lung cancer. More generally, perhaps the best explanation for causal regularities is that there are necessary connections between causes and effects after all (in other words, contrary to Hume, we have good reason to believe in necessary connection *in the objects*).

Inference to the best explanation is a form of inductive reasoning, at least insofar as (i) the conclusions drawn are *matters of fact* inferred from empirical evidence, and (ii) that there is no logical contradiction in supposing those conclusions might turn out to be false. In short, if inference to the best explanation is a justified mode of reasoning, at least *some* inductive inferences are justified.

Although inference to the best explanation is on the face of it appealing, it too has its problems. Van Fraassen has argued that there is often more than one theory compatible with a set of empirical data, so we need a *principle of privilege* to choose between the competing theories [169]. Further, even if we *can* choose the best of the available hypotheses, and even if the best explanation is true, it is possible that all of the competing theories we have are false. How can we know that the true hypothesis – the hypothesis that best explains the phenomenon – is included in our set of competing hypotheses? Unless we can know this, inference to the best explanation does not look to be a fully justified method of inference.

4.3.2.3 The Pragmatic Solution

Blaise Pascal (1623–62) once argued that it is rational to live one's life as if God exists, and one should endeavour to believe in His existence. Unlike arguments such as the cosmological and ontological arguments for the existence of God, "Pascal's wager" is purely pragmatic. He argues that we are betting with our lives: if one lives one's life as if God exists, the potential losses are finite (no tennis on a Sunday morning), and the potential gains infinite (an eternity of happiness in Heaven). If one fails to live one's life as if God exists then the potential gains are finite (tennis on Sunday morning), but the potential losses infinite (an eternity in Hell). So it is rational to live one's life as if God exists [337].

A similar strategy can be employed to argue for the rationality of induction. Here, too, we are "betting with our lives". Nature has, thus far, been uniform: the Sun has always risen in the East, all observed electrons have had charge −1, stepping out the window of a 5 storey building had always ended badly, and so on. We can either bet on the rationality of induction, and assume that Nature will continue to be uniform in this way, or we can behave as if all inductive inferences are unjustified (such that we may as well step out of the 5 story building). We *may* live in a world where Nature turns out not to be uniform, in which case our inductions will fail whether we take induction to be rational or not. But we may (and hopefully do) live in a world where Nature will always be uniform. In this world, when we correctly identify causal relationships, our everyday inductions will (mostly) succeed. So we may as well behave as if inductive reasoning is rational.

The history of medicine is rife with examples of failed inductions. Hypotheses concerning the causes of disease and curative/preventative interventions have consistently been refuted, and entire medical paradigms have been overturned. But betting that empirical evidence can in principle lead us to the true causes of disease, and help us correctly identify curative and preventative interventions, is our only hope, so we *must* take at least some inductions to be rational. This leaves us with the problem of "which inductions are rational?" In the case of medicine, this boils down to how to identify true causal relationships over mere associations.

4.4 Epidemiology and Identifying Causation

Arguably the core competency of epidemiologists is to identify causes and causal interventions, and specifically distinguishing causal regularities from mere associations. As we have already discussed, a variety of statistical methods are used to achieve this goal, primarily comprising various forms of clinical trials. Outside of the domain of medical research, the identification of causal connections is also fundamental for the clinician (whether a general practitioner, cardiologist, oncologist, orthopaedic surgeon…). We have seen that inductive inferences are fallible, and have considered arguments suggesting that causation is not directly observable, so how can those working in the medical sciences legitimately practice their profession? In this section we look at several strategies, focusing on the epidemiologist, and consider how successful/reliable these strategies are given the problems we have already identified.

4.4.1 The Potential Outcomes Approach Revisited

In the previous chapter we discussed the POA in relation to the counterfactual account of singular causation. We concluded that although there were similarities insofar as causation is identified by comparing observed events with unobservable, counterfactual events, they fundamentally differ insofar as the POA is designed to provide general causal claims such as "smoking causes cancer", rather than singular causal claims such as "smoking caused Jane's cancer". Although identifying singular causation is extremely important for clinicians, the identification of singular causation in clinical practice is typically dependent on medical knowledge of more general causal claims. If we did not know that "smoking causes cancer", then it would be far more difficult for the clinician to point at "smoking" as the cause of Jane's cancer. If the potential outcomes approach is successful, it is an invaluable tool in public health.

Remember that the POA requires data from only one *actual* intervention. The remaining data necessary for the strategy comes from "contrary-to-fact" interventions, such that one measures the causal effect of the actual intervention by comparing the actual data with that from the contrary-to-fact interventions. Given the counterfactual account of causation discussed in Chap. 3, this strategy looks plausible. The primary theoretical problem, however, is that it depends heavily upon the accuracy of the contrary-to-fact data. By definition, it is logically impossible to be sure that the data used from the contrary-to-fact intervention is what we would really get were the contrary-to-fact intervention the actual intervention, since one cannot simultaneously use both interventions. Further, even if we *could* guarantee the accuracy of our counterfactual data, there is no guarantee that the actual data would generalise; that is to say, the problem of induction could always strike.

4.4.2 Observational Studies and Randomised Controlled Trials

Observational studies and randomised controlled trials suffer much the same general problem as the POA. Case control studies and cohort studies compare groups of participants over a period of time, but just as there was no way of knowing for sure whether the child nutrition project in Tamil Nadu would be successful in Bangladesh, so there is no way of guaranteeing that *any* observational study is generalizable. Similarly, even if the randomization strategies used by RCTs show that the intervention under investigation was a "difference-maker" within that specific trial, this does not prove with certainty that the same intervention will make a difference in future trials, or in the patients that will ultimately use the treatments as curative/preventative measures.

The first problem with the POA stems from the logical impossibility of knowing the outcomes of contrary-to-fact studies, but the POA, observational studies and RCTs all fall foul to the problem of induction. That being said, the pragmatic solution to the problem of induction arguably nevertheless justifies using the interventions developed through clinical trials when treating patients.

In this section we have looked at three methods used by epidemiologists to identify causal relationships, but we have not yet considered whether a coherent set of more general viewpoints can be set out to distinguish causal relationships from mere associations. These can be understood as heuristics that aid in decision making. Used in this way, the heuristics work in a binary fashion: If they are present, i.e., if they are a characteristic of a certain risk factor, then the risk factor is a cause. The Henle-Koch view of individual causes leading to individual diseases has led to the concept of causal inference by "criteria", such as those put forward by Sir Austin Bradford Hill [32]. This will be the focus of the next section.

4.5 Hill's Heuristics

According to a popular internet search engine (accessed on May 15, 2014), Hill's "Environment and disease – association or causation" has been cited 5619 times since its publication half a century ago [32]. We think this justifies its characterization as one of the more successful pieces in the epidemiologic literature.

4.5.1 *Association or Causation?*

In January 1965, Sir Austin Bradford Hill delivered his President's Address before the Occupational Medicine Section of the Royal Society of Medicine [32]. His title was *The Environment and Disease: Association or Causation*. At the beginning of his lecture, Hill asks "in what circumstances can we pass from (an) observed association to a verdict of causation?" Moreover, he asks, "How do we detect relationships between sickness, injury and conditions of work?" and goes on to propose nine "aspects of that association [we should] consider before deciding that the most likely interpretation of it is causation". In essence, Hill was interested in exploring which aspects of an apparent association between a risk factor and disease should be considered when making decisions about the likelihood of working at a causal relation.

Hill offered two potentially helpful concepts.

First, he cautiously defined a cause within his framework of environmental medicine as a change in an environmental feature A that influences the frequency of an undesirable event B. In a way, Bunge's view of causation "as a (or even the) way events are generated" (see preface to the 1979 Dover edition of [8]).

Second, Hill came up with discussion points ("criteria" in Henle/Koch thinking), that ask for an evaluation of the strength of the relationship between a cause and its effect, its consistency (repeated observations by different investigators in different populations etc.), specificity, temporality, biological gradient, plausibility, coherence, experiment, and analogy. After discussing each single one, Hill states "Here then are nine different viewpoints from all of which we should study association before we cry causation."

Towards the end of his paper, Hill alluded to the idea that the heuristics he just developed should not be used as if they were hard-and-fast criteria and adds the caveat that "none can bring indisputable evidence for or against the cause and effect hypothesis and none can be required a sine qua non."

4.5.2 *Hill Discussed*

Hill's criteria have been discussed to a great extent in epidemiology. An early critic of criteria, Rothman [27] suggests that other than the fixed time order of cause and effect "there are no reliable criteria for determining whether an association is causal." A decade later, Rothman and Greenland's perception has not changed considerably [95]. Weed suggests a "Popperian alternative to Hill's criteria" [170]. He shows that Hill's criteria cannot be deducted fully to support/reject hypotheses of sufficient cause, necessary cause, and disease process. He suggests as new criteria predictability and testability. He goes on to discuss the ontological, methodological and ethical problems of cause and concludes that "the scientific process never ends up with certain knowledge about cause". As replacement for certainty he discusses the pros and cons of belief, probability, and criticism.

This concept has been criticized by many. Phillips and Goodman [171] suggest that *criteria* such as Hill's should be called *considerations*. (Hill himself wrote that his suggestions are NOT criteria; he called them *viewpoints*.) Poole [172] prefers to call them "values", which is a fantastic way of making very clear that criteria are not objective and are probably best viewed not as structured like a binary yes/no variable, but as a somewhat wobbly more/less variable.

In essence, the postulation of criteria such as Hill's is nothing but a replacement of one dilemma with another: why should it be easier to identify the truth condition of the criteria than identifying the truth condition of the relationship between exposure and effect? In fact, the very idea to develop criteria for causal inference does not seem pragmatic at all. What might be pragmatist (i.e., Jamesian or Deweyian) would be asking the question differently, i.e., how can we identify causes in a way that makes our lives a little better? Since there is not much room for absolute reference in pragmatism, the identification of causation does not make much sense beyond enabling us to act upon them in order to improve the human condition. Indeed, without absolute reference, the entire concept of verification, and falsification for that matter [101], seems difficult beyond the comparison of criteria to gold standards, which are notoriously soft in nature and can misdirect if wrong [102]. The very notion of criteria encapsulates the view of "if, and only if", which is in itself deterministic lingo and concept par excellence, pointing at necessary causes only, not at unnecessary causes or sufficient causal constellations.

Since Hill called them *viewpoints* or *aspects*, his language suggests that he considered them subjective, his own perspective. Indeed, Hill wrote that "none of my nine viewpoints can bring indisputable evidence for or against the cause-and-effect hypothesis and none can be required as a sine qua non" ([32], italics in original). Others, however, have called Hill's characteristics *criteria* [99, 173]. By taking this position, perhaps they suggest that it might somehow be possible to use them as such.

The story of how Hill came to write his viewpoints in 1965 is interesting in its own right, but too convoluted to be exhibited here in its full glory. As told by Henry Blackburn and Darwin Labarthe, the genesis of Hill's viewpoints was based on exchanges among scientists during the decade before Hill published his paper; their paper gives proper credit to scholars who made extensive intellectual contributions to the development of Hill's viewpoints: Ancel Keys, Herman Hilleboe, Jacob Yerushalmy, Carroll Palmer, Abraham Lilienfeld, Philip Sartwell, Cuyler Hammond, Reuel Stallone, Alfredo Morabia, and Sir Austin Bradford Hill himself [174].

Today, Hill's viewpoints are considered the sui generis epidemiologic approach to causal inference. Indeed, Morabia compared David Hume's and John Stuart Mill's thoughts and Hill's viewpoints and concludes that Hill cannot be derived directly from these two authors' thinking [106].

4.5.3 Debunking Soft Criterianism

Despite all theorizing about the possibility and the current prevailing perception that disease causation does not lend itself to inference-by-criterion, most epidemiologists concede that somehow, associations that fulfill more of Hill's "criteria" are more likely to be causal than associations that fulfill fewer. Here, we show that even this "soft criterianism" is unfounded. In this section, we respond to each one of Hill's nine viewpoints, trying to refute each single one. Each viewpoint comes with a verbatim quote from Lucas & MacMichael [175], who provide a brief explanation.

> **Strength**. Bradford Hill suggested that strong associations were more likely to be causal than weak associations.

Why should "strong associations" be more likely to be causal than weak ones? How would you support such claim? You would need to analyze a large dataset, identify strong and weak associations, however defined, and show that significantly more of the strong associations are actually causal compared to the weak ones. How can you do that, if you don't know how to establish causality in the first place?

Nothing inherent to odds ratios or risk ratios indicates the likelihood of this effect measure to be causal. All these numbers indicate are, well, the strength of the association. This is what Alex Broadbent has called "the causal interpretation problem" [80]. He writes, "the mathematical definition of the measures in question do not answer these questions: they do not tell us how to understand the causal import of a measure of association on those occasions when it is used to express a causal fact, as well as a fact about an association" [80].

> **Consistency**. Bradford Hill also felt more confidence in a causal explanation for an association if the same answer had been achieved in a variety of different situations — prospectively and retrospectively and in different populations.

Again, why should consistency increase credibility of a causal claim? Yes, it makes intuitive sense, but do we not think, since Hume, that no number of observations justifies the prediction of the next one with certainty? Did not Popper argue rather cogently that no number of observations of white swans justifies the conclusion that all swans are white? Nothing unique to multiple observations excludes the possibility that even a large number of repetitive successes of a new drug in a string of RCTs might be a chance event.

> **Specificity**. This criterion is often stated to mean that any exposure may give rise to only a single outcome (13). While this may be true for some infectious diseases, for example only rubella virus causes rubella, it is clearly unlikely with respect to many environmental exposures. Bradford Hill recognized that diseases may have more than one cause and that one-to-one relationships are not frequent. However, if an association is limited to specific groups with a particular environmental exposure or is greatly increased in these groups, then the case for a causal association is strengthened.

Apparently, Hill himself realized the weakness of the idea of specificity. In its purest form, specificity means that "only cause C causes only effect E". Indeed, a rare thing in epidemiology and medicine. The idea probably comes from the Koch/Henle postulates, which were intended for infectious disease research, but is marginally helpful in chronic disease epidemiology, which champions a multicausal [33] and multiple possible outcomes scenario.

> **Temporality**. Temporality is a necessary criterion for a causal association between an exposure and an outcome, that is, the exposure must precede the outcome.

This one is the least interesting characteristic, because it appears to be a tautology, exemplified by the common knowledge that we cannot go backward in time.

This, in turn, is just so because we define time as moving forward, never backwards. Thus, the process of causation must go forward, by definition. Should we ever reach agreement that the *delayed quantum choice experiment* by Kim and colleagues [176] has indeed shown that photons can retroactively change their choice whether to be a wave or a particle backward in time, the temporality characteristic will change from truism to invalid claim. Neither is helpful in deciding whether an association is causal or not.

> **Biological gradient**. It seems logical that the likelihood of a causal association is increased if a biological gradient or dose–response curve can be demonstrated.

Many biological mechanisms appear to exhibit a threshold effect-behavior; with increasing "dosage of exposure" we see only small changes in outcome until a threshold is reached. At this point, an appreciable and sudden change of magnitude in the outcome occurs without any (or very little) change in exposure dosage. Yes, this is sort of a dose-response as well, but it is not steady and can be difficult to detect.

> **Plausibility**. While it is reassuring if a causal association is biologically plausible, Bradford Hill notes that "this is a feature I am convinced we cannot demand.

Even if we cannot demand plausibility, does its availability increase the likelihood of causality? Yes, if the additional data that make the causal claim more likely are solid in themselves. But how do we know that? If the reference data make the same claim as the exposure-outcome dyad whose causality is in question, how do we establish their causality. Seems a little bit like robbing Peter to pay Paul?

> **Coherence**. Coherence and biological plausibility share a requirement that the cause-and-effect interpretation of an association should fit with the known facts of the natural history and biology of the disease.

Indeed. Vide supra, our comment on *plausibility*.

> **Experiment**. Do preventive actions taken on the basis of a demonstrated cause-and-effect association alter the frequency of the outcome? With overtones of Koch's postulates, this criterion offered, in Bradford Hill's view, the strongest support of a causal interpretation.

Some may think that experimental laboratory work can indeed reveal true causation. However, as much as laboratory studies allow the experimenter to control many or even all potentially confounding or biasing factors, the unique experimental scenario comes with uncertain applicability to the real-life, human system. Still, some think that "the strength of the randomized experiment is its capacity to facilitate the causal inference that change A caused a change in the probability that B would occur. However, one of the oldest criticisms of the randomized experiment is that it is so locally defined that this clear causal inference comes at the cost of one's inability to generalize the causal connection found" [177](p.341) Ken Rothman and Sander Greenland appear to agree when they write that

> Some experimental scientists hold that epidemiologic relations are only suggestive and believe that detailed the laboratory study of mechanisms within single individuals can reveal cause–effect relations with certainty. This view overlooks the fact that all relations are suggested in

> exactly the manner discussed by Hume: Even the most careful and detailed mechanistic dissection of individual events cannot provide more than associations, albeit at a finer level. [95]

Unfortunately, the same is true in epidemiology. As we have already claimed, even RCTs cannot prove causation. John Worrall summarizes his view after having discussed the epistemological value of RCTs in general and randomization in particular, as follows:

> All trial results are defeasible. We are always, quite trivially, at the mercy of the possibility that the two groups are, unbeknown to us, unbalanced in some significant way. And, whatever may be true in the theoretical indefinite long run of endlessly repeated random divisions, for real-world trials, randomization does exactly nothing to alleviate this worry (remember selection bias is a 'known' factor). The best we can do (as ever) is test our theories against rivals that seem plausible in the light of background knowledge. Once we have eliminated other explanations that we know are possible (by suitable deliberate, or post hoc, control) we have done as much as we can epistemologically. The unthinking pursuit of randomization in all circumstances seems simply to be bad epistemology. [178]

Back to Hill.

> **Analogy.** Bradford Hill and other epidemiologists recognized that the notion of analogy can be taken to impractical extremes and may depend on the imagination of scientists to see analogies. Clear-cut analogies, however, may add to the weight of evidence for otherwise weak associations.

So what is analogy? How clear-cut does the analogy need to be to be counted as having the potential to add to the weight of evidence? Is it sufficient to find epidemiologic evidence? Another study that shows an analogous association, in an error-independent way? How many factors need to be kept constant? Exposure only? Outcome only? Neither, and similar exposures/outcomes would count? Or is method-independent evidence needed? For example, do we need animal experiments in which mice are exposed to cigarette smoke and are observed over time with regard to cardiopulmonary consequences? Some of us think that experimental and epidemiologic evidence together make a pretty strong case in favor of causation. Others think that "the cliché that epidemiologic studies generate only measures of association, not causation is meaningless... even experiments just generate measures of association as well" [28]. If experimental evidence, are mice sufficiently close to the human system under investigation, or do we need evidence from larger animals? Rats? Pigs? Primates? Above and beyond method independence this would offer species independence as well. Who decides?

4.6 Gold Standard?

As if the above deconstruction of all nine of Hill's viewpoints was not enough, there is one additional issue that makes it difficult to understand their popularity if not as criteria then as probability of causation increasers. This additional issue is related to the apparent lack of a Gold Standard that could be used as a reference point for the decision that the likelihood of the association under investigation being indeed causal is increased.

Some of Hill's viewpoints have, indirectly, been rejected previously by P.R. Burch, a dauntless crusader against the idea that smoking might cause lung cancer [179]. Burch discussed in 1983 his concerns about the five causal criteria used in a report on "Smoking and health" written by a committee appointed by the U.S. Surgeon General [180], which were likely part of the basis for Hill's paper [174]. Burch writes

> not one of the criteria, plausibly interpreted, is satisfied by the epidemiologic evidence for lung cancer. A weakness underlying all the Reports is a prior failure to recognize all the logical possibilities inherent in an association between smoking and a disease. The five criteria and the subjective method of "judgment" are inappropriate to a scientific analysis; they should be replaced by the objective testing of hypotheses.

He concludes that "the entire association between cigarette smoking and lung cancer [...] is unlikely to be explained by causation." Despite the fact that Burch's conclusion is highly likely false, his points about the criteria and the "judgment – issue" are well taken. Indeed, current textbook wisdom has that "Hill himself was ambivalent about the utility of these 'standards' [...] and disagreed that any 'hard – and – fast rules of evidence' existed by which to judge causation" [95]. Ken Rothman and Sander Greenland consider Hill's fourth viewpoint, temporality, "a sine qua non for causality" [95]. Still, they hold that "there is no necessary or sufficient criterion for determining whether an observed association is causal" [95].

If asked whether he would strongly believe that an association that fulfils all of his 'criteria' is indeed causal, even if he cannot be absolutely certain, we believe that Hill would have answered "Yes". Therefore, we suggest we are justified in assuming that, for Hill, the summa of all nine of his "criteria" was nothing more or less as his definition of disease causation. And we also think that most of us would agree. Which means that we appear to have some kind of *silver standard*, which does not provide an absolute reference point, but a relative one; one that is good enough for all intents and purposes. What could this silver standard be? A silver standard will require to be defined in a non-deterministic, probabilistic way as that what, being modified, is regularly associated with a change in occurrence, severity, or outcomes of disease. This strips Hill's *criteria* of their status as truth-makers and allows them to be *viewpoints* from which to look at the silver standard and using them as *quasi-criteria* for causal reasoning, perhaps even inference.

The postulation of criteria such as Hill's is nothing but a replacement of one dilemma with another: why should it be easier to identify the truth condition of the criteria than identifying the truth criteria of the relationship between exposure and effect right before our very eyes? In fact, the very idea to develop criteria for causal inference does not seem pragmatic at all. A pragmatist (i.e., Jamesian or Deweyian philosopher) would ask the question differently, i.e., how can we identify causes in a way that makes our lives a little better? Since there is not much room for absolute reference in pragmatism, the identification of causation does not make much sense beyond enabling us to act upon them in order to improve the human condition.

4.7 Is There Such a Thing as Medical Knowledge?

Before one answers the question "is there medical knowledge?" one must make clear what it is to know something; a conceptual analysis of knowledge must be adopted. A thorough investigation of contemporary epistemology is well beyond the scope of this book, so here we provide just a brief discussion. We argue that medical knowledge is possible under at least one analysis, despite the inescapable fallibility of our causal inferences.

4.7.1 The Tripartite Account of Knowledge

In Sect. 4.2.2 we mentioned the Platonic, tripartite conception of knowledge as "justified true belief" (JTB), according to which an agent S knows proposition P if and only if:

1. S believes that P
2. S is justified in believing that P
3. P is true

This conception is problematic, since it is possible to satisfy all three conditions without knowing P. Consider the following example (adapted from [181]):

Sam is trying for a baby. She uses the home pregnancy test she bought in the pharmacy, and it is positive. This justifies Sam's belief that "Sam is pregnant (A)". If Sam's belief that she is pregnant is justified, then she is justified in believing any disjunctive proposition that includes A as a disjunct. Sam is thus justified in believing that "either Sam is pregnant or Sam has cancer" (A or B) (that she has no reason to believe she has cancer is irrelevant). Now suppose that Sam's pregnancy test was a false positive (A is false), but Sam does in fact have cancer (B is true). Where "S" is Sam, A is "Sam is pregnant", and B is "Sam has cancer",

1. S believes that "A or B"
2. S is justified in believing that "A or B"
3. "A or B" is true

Sam's belief that "A or B" is true in virtue of B, and justified by the positive pregnancy test. According to the JTB account of knowledge, then, Sam knows that "either she is pregnant or she has cancer". But this would be a strange claim, since the source of justification and the fact that makes the proposition true are entirely unrelated. "Justified true belief" is thus widely regarded as (at best) insufficient for knowledge, so a number of alternative theories have been offered. We discuss one such theory, the causal theory of knowing [182], below.

4.7.2 Internalism, Externalism, and the KK Principle

The tripartite account of knowledge is what philosophers call an *internalist* account of knowledge (note that despite the failure of JTB, there are motivations for being an internalist) [183]. According to internalism, the *warrant* that distinguishes true belief from knowledge is internal to our cognitive perspective: one can see whether one's beliefs are warranted through reflection and introspection. Externalists, on the other hand, take what warrants beliefs to lie external to one's cognitive perspective.

Internalists tend to endorse what is commonly known as the KK principle: the principle that in order to know that P, one must be in a position to know that one knows it [184]. This makes sense for the internalist, since internalists consider themselves to be in a position to know whether one's beliefs are warranted (and knowing that one knows P, in addition to P being true, is mainly a matter of knowing that one's belief that P is warranted). Externalists generally reject the principle, however, since if the warrant for P is external to the agent, it is quite possible for the agent not to be in position to know that their belief that P is warranted.

The discussion of the problem of induction and the examples from the history of medicine highlighted how fallible our "medical knowledge" is. Indeed, it would be fair to say that we rarely (if ever) know that we know our medical beliefs, despite the evidence we may have for them. According to the KK principle, it seems that medical knowledge is not genuine knowledge.

4.7.3 Externalism to the Rescue: The Causal Theory of Knowing

There are a number of externalist theories of knowledge that try to improve on JTB, including (but not restricted to) *reliabilism* [185] and *the causal theory of knowing* [182]. The reliabilist believes that in order one to know that P, the *belief that P* must have been produced by a reliable process; but of course an agent's belief can be produced by a reliable process she is ignorant of, making it impossible for her to know that she knows that P. Reliabilists thus reject the KK principle.

For simplicity's sake, we shall focus on Goldman's causal theory of knowing, and argue that medical knowledge *as genuine knowledge* is possible after all.

Recognising the shortfalls in the tripartite account, Alvin Goldman introduced a causal condition to his analysis of knowledge, such that "S knows that p if and only if the fact p is causally connected in an "appropriate" way with S's believing p" [182:364].

In the example above, Sam's belief that P ("either Sam is pregnant or Sam has cancer") is not causally connected *in an appropriate way* to the fact that P, so it would not count as knowledge. But now consider the claim "smoking causes cancer" (if anything counts as medical knowledge it is this). If smoking *does* cause cancer, then this fact is responsible for the significant results of the clinical trials.

The results of those trials caused the medical profession to accept the causal connection between smoking and cancer. Given that the causal relation is transitive (if A causes B, and B causes C, then A causes C), there is a causal chain between the fact that smoking caused cancer in the participants, and our belief that smoking causes cancer. Since smoking does in fact cause cancer (P is true), according to the causal account "smoking causes cancer" is a genuine case of knowledge.

To sum up, for the externalist, the fact that we cannot be sure of the causal connection is irrelevant (we don't know that we know). What matters is the metaphysical issue of there *being* a causal connection between the fact that *smoking causes cancer* and our belief that *smoking causes cancer*, not the epistemological question of whether we know that there really is a causal connection between the two. It turns out that the difficulties we encountered regarding identifying causation in public health do not necessarily preclude us from having medical knowledge. It's just that what we take to be medical knowledge is fallible.

4.8 Wrapping Up

In this chapter we considered how a number of core philosophy debates apply to the fundamental goals of population health. In particular, how the problem of induction and related difficulties in identifying causal relationships feature so prominently in our ability to claim genuine medical knowledge. We argued in the final section that medical knowledge *qua* knowledge is possible, but one cannot, and should not claim that what we take to be medical knowledge is infallible.

Ultimately, those propositions we take to be medical facts can only be known if they are true, and as philosophers such as Hume have demonstrated (and as history attests) there is no guarantee that the causal relationships we readily accept are anything more than mere associations. If we deny the KK principle, though, we are in principle capable of having genuine medical knowledge – but we can never know which of our medical knowledge claims are genuine cases of knowledge.

The pragmatic solution to the problem of induction tells us that we should believe that nature is uniform – largely because it's our only option – and so the question becomes which associations should we take to be causal. Which medical theories should we endorse? Medicine has provided us with a number of answers to this question: carefully-designed studies, despite regularly being falsified, provide us with at least some evidence for genuine causal relationships, and although we find his position unconvincing, the heuristics provided by Bradford-Hill is an attempt to do the same. But ultimately, regardless of how successful these strategies may be, it is only prudent never to take a theory to be confirmed; rather adopt the Popperian strategy of continually testing the *medical knowledge* claims we tentatively endorse, with a view to proving them false.

Chapter 5
Making Population Health Knowledge

Abstract This chapter revolves around the idea that knowledge is generated from data. We briefly describe Ackoff's hierarchy, which starts with data and proceeds via information to knowledge, understanding and wisdom. In contrast, we propose to de-emphasize understanding and wisdom, and to insert evidence between information and knowledge. We outline a framework that takes data as raw symbols, which morph into information when contextualized. Information becomes evidence when compared to relevant standards. Evidence is used to test hypotheses and is transformed into knowledge by consensus. As quality checkpoints for the transition between levels we offer relevance, robustness, repeatability, and reproducibility.

Keywords Data · Information · Evidence · Knowledge · Context · Comparison · Consensus

5.1 Introduction

Data, information, and knowledge are central concepts in informatics and data science. The transition from data to knowledge is not exactly straightforward. There are no formal rules, and sometimes not even good definitions for the concepts involved. In this chapter, we outline the reasoning process that generates knowledge from raw data.

In our target scenario (Fig. 1.1 in Chap. 1), the three concepts have a prominent place (in the top right corner box) as the readouts to be expected from Public Health Information Systems: from the causal web of population health phenomena and from health system performance monitoring. But what exactly does it mean, to *gather data*, to *obtain information*, and to *generate knowledge*?

Consider the following two quotes:

> One major goal of public health informatics is ensuring the capacity to assess community problems in a comprehensive manner through the development of integrated nationwide public health data systems. This will require a clear definition of public health data needs

---

We borrow the title of this chapter from Miriam Solomon's book, *Making Medical Knowledge,* [186].

O. Dammann, B. Smart, *Causation in Population Health Informatics and Data Science*, https://doi.org/10.1007/978-3-319-96307-5_5

> and the sources for these data, consensus on data and communications standards—to facilitate data quality, comparability and exchange—along with policies to support data sharing and mechanisms and tools for accessing and disseminating data and information in a useful manner. [187]

> The literature consistently indicated a critical need for comprehensive, coordinated, and accessible information to meet the needs of the public health workforce. Major barriers to information access include time, resource reliability, trustworthiness/credibility of information, and 'information overload' [...] There is a critical need for public health digital knowledge management systems designed to reflect the diversity of public health activities, to enable human communications, and to provide multiple access points to critical information resources. Public health librarians and other information specialists can serve a significant role in helping public health professionals meet their information needs through the development of evidence-based decision support systems, human-mediated expert searching and training in the use information retrieval systems. [188]

In this chapter, we first discuss the hierarchy proposed by organizational theorist Russell L. Ackoff (1919–2009) in 1989 [189]. Subsequently, we offer our own version, which discards Ackoff's notion of *wisdom*, making room for the notion of *evidence*.

5.2 The Knowledge Pyramid

5.2.1 Ackoff's Hierarchy

Russell L. Ackoff (1919–2009) is often credited with being the father of the so-called *knowledge hierarchy* or *knowledge pyramid* (Fig. 5.1). Ackoff was an academic operations and management scientist.[1] His knowledge pyramid paper was not really a scientific treatise, but more of an opinion piece, given as the presidential address to the International Society for General Systems Research (ISGSR) in 1988 [189]. In the published version, Ackoff suggests the following relationships between data, information, knowledge and wisdom.

Ackoff starts with the notion that wisdom is situated at the top of a hierarchy of types of content in the mind, followed by understanding, knowledge, information, and data [189:3] (Fig. 5.1; of note, the original article does not have a figure, nor does it refer to pryamids.) He defines *data* as symbols that are properties of observables, and *information* as descriptions. Ackoff sees the difference between the two not as structural, but functional, and information as inferred from data. In a discussion of management needs in terms of information availability, he states that managers face an information overload and do not necessarily need more relevant information, but less irrelevant information. Next, Ackoff defines *knowledge* as know-how that, so he wrote, comes from learning, i.e., by instruction or from experience, and adaptation, i.e., the correction of the learned in accordance with new circumstances. One notion

[1] https://www.informs.org/Explore/History-and-Traditions/Biographical-Profiles/Ackoff-Russell-L; accessed 4/7/2017.

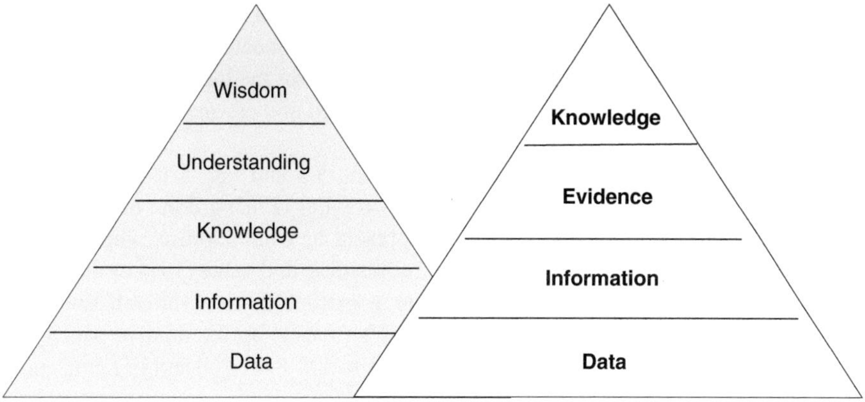

Fig. 5.1 Ackoff's knowledge hierarchy (left) and our proposed modification (right)

of Ackoff's that is rather important in the present context is that this process requires understanding error, why error occurs, and how to correct it.

At this point, Ackoff introduces *efficiency* and *effectiveness* and states that this distinction (which he does not define exactly) differentiates wisdom from intelligence, the latter being reflected in our capacity to understand based on knowledge and information. He says that wisdom is *the ability to increase* effectiveness, while *intelligence is the ability to increase efficiency*. Again, Ackoff does not exactly define efficiency and effectiveness, but offers growth and development as a parallel construct, where *growth* does not imply an increase in value, while *development* does.

In the remainder of his paper, Ackoff goes into more depth about ethical issues and into an incursion into classical philosophy, referring to Plato and Aristotle, a philosophical reference without direct bearing on our discussion. The bottom lines of his paper are (1) that information systems can be automated and generate information out of data, (2) that computer-based knowledge systems require higher-order mental faculties; "they do not develop knowledge, but apply knowledge developed by people", and (3) that wisdom adds value, endures forever, and will probably never be generated by machines.

5.2.2 *Wisdom or Knowledge?*

As outlined above, Ackoff's hierarchy is often depicted as a triangle or pyramid (as we do in Fig. 5.1). With data representing the foundation, the hierarchy ascends via information and knowledge, towards wisdom at the pinnacle. Jennifer Rowley has suggested calling the concept the "wisdom hierarchy" [190]. Although she seems more interested in wisdom than in other components of the pyramid, the main part of her 2007 paper is a summary of terminological definitions, of *data, information, knowledge, and wisdom*, as pulled from major textbooks used in information system and knowledge management education. Her review reiterates two opinions; first, her view that data, information, and knowledge are connected, one helping define the other, and second, her view about the organization of the hierarchy as such. The nature of the ways how the three things are converted and elevated to the next level is less well defined.

Our version of the hierarchy (see below, Sect. 5.3 and Fig. 5.1, on right) will propose a system of transitions that is based on what is being done to make such transitions possible, not what transitions represent or what happens when moving from one level to another, such as changes of meaning and value [191] or the physical, cognitive, and belief structuring when constructing data, information, and knowledge, respectively [192]. Again, Rowley's focus is on the relative paucity of explications of *wisdom*. Our focus is instead the fact that the concept of *knowledge*, which is at the top of our hierarchy, is not well defined either.

A similar model has been proposed by Richard Heller (Heller 2005:84). In his model, accessing data yields information, appraisal of which yields knowledge. What is missing in Heller's model is the distinct role that evidence plays between information and knowledge (see our model below). Neither in his book [116] nor in the underlying paper [193] does Heller define evidence. However, in their 2002 paper, Heller and Page offer a list of statistical and implementation characteristics they see as methods with an appropriate population focus that can be aligned with the methods used in evidence-based medicine because the authors consider the entire process from data via information to knowledge to be *evidence-generating*.

5.3 DIEK: Data, Information, Evidence, Knowledge

We suggest dropping wisdom from our system for two reasons. First, the term is fraught with too much baggage from non-scientific context. Second, we disagree with Ackoff's somewhat shallow definition of wisdom as the addition of value to knowledge that requires judgement. In contrast, we believe that judgement is part of the process at all levels of transition in the hierarchy. We do not think that wisdom adds to the decision-making based on the hierarchy, perhaps with a few exceptions when decisions are made in which stakeholders consider it prudent to go beyond scientific considerations. In contrast, we think that knowledge is a fine endpoint of the ascending hierarchy. We believe that knowledge is well-prepared for its role as pinnacle of the triangle when we define it, in our context of medical and public health data science, as *predictive, testable, consistently successful belief*, as long as there is a causal connection between the facts represented by the data, information, and evidence on the one hand, and our beliefs on the other.

Within the domain of causal explanation, we propose a specific manner for interpreting the levels of this hierarchy. The distinction between data and information may be understood as that between sample data and the probability distribution that is estimated from those data, respectively. While there are many forms of data interpretation that play a role in causal inference, the use of statistical methods to infer features of a probability distribution is especially important. When we ask whether two correlated variables are *causally* related, we presuppose that these variables are in fact *associated*, and this *association* must be inferred from the sample. Moving on, the relationship between knowledge and information may be understood as that between a causal model and a probability distribution. While the probability distribution provides information that enables one to predict the values of variables conditional on those of other variables, the correct causal model provides knowledge of which variables may be changed by intervening on other variables [70, 194]. Causal knowledge is thus essential for health interventions and policy. Yet knowledge that one variable causes another only indicates that there are some interventions by which one can use the former to influence the latter.

5.3.1 Data Are Data Are Data

In the context of Public Health Informatics, Mensah and Goderre describe "data" as raw facts, statistics, context-free numbers [195]. We'd like to take a more general position and suggest that data are numbers, symbols, and text as retrieved, collected, or simulated (Table 5.1). Data are typically generated in the form of measurements of physical entities, results of experiments, text-mining, census data, surveys, simulations, etc. They can be tabulated and depicted as graphs, or displayed as figures.

Table 5.1 Characteristics of data, information, evidence, and knowledge

CONCEPT	What is it?	How produced?	By whom?	With what goal?
Data	Numbers Symbols Text Unit values	**Collection from** Field research, Database Measurements in experiments, individuals, or populations	Data collector (multiple job descriptions)	Use as raw data Use for information generation Storage, curation, retrieval
Information	Data In context	**Contextualization by** Making data useful for, and using them for specific tasks	Informatician, Informaticist, Statistician	Use as source for Answering questions Storage, curation, retrieval,
Evidence	Useful, contextualized information	**Comparison with** Standards Reference values Reference information	Scientist, Philosopher	Use for analyses designed to support specific claims/hypotheses, e.g., in scientific publications
Knowledge	Solid information, (e.g., passed the 5R Test)	**Consensus** based on Reasoning, Discussion	Scientist, Philosopher	Justification of health interventions

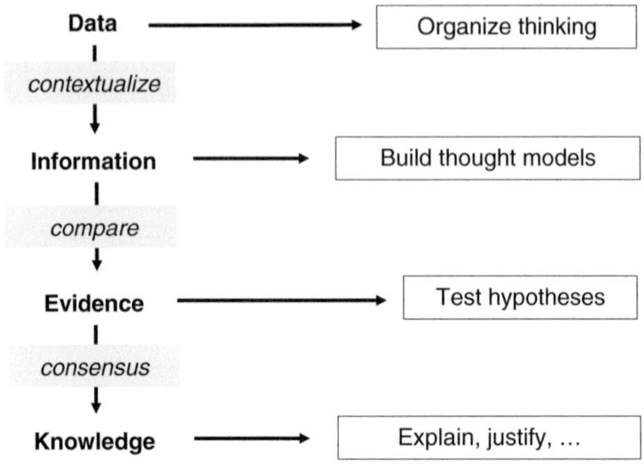

Fig. 5.2 Suggested framework for transition from data to knowledge (winged arrows), and what it is good for (straight arrows)

More formally speaking, data are quantitative or qualitative expressions of variables.

Definition *Data* are numbers, symbols, and text as retrieved, collected, or simulated.

Take, for example, the numbers 50 and 1000. These numbers not represent much, perhaps only that one is smaller than the other and that both are divisible by 2, 5, 10 etc. Once we add "km" to the first and "degrees Fahrenheit" to the other, we know that the first is a measure of length or distance, and the second a temperature. This is meaningful data.

The current buzzword *Big Data* refers to data generated by large data collection systems with very wide, sometimes global reach, for example the raw data collected by social media platforms and patient information stored in the databases of large insurance companies. Once such large databases are linked, they provide *information*. Indeed, the mere motivation for the database merger provides context that, in our view, transforms data into information.

In Fig. 5.2, we propose a framework for transitions from data to knowledge, and what the arrival at each new stage is good for. We will come back to quality checkpoints for these transitions in Sect. 5.4.

5.3.2 *Information Is Data Contextualized*

Mensah & Goderre further suggest that "information is the collection, aggregation, analysis, and presentation of data that provides understanding" [195]. We think that this definition describes how we arrive at information based on data, but does not say much about what information *is*. We offer the following definition:

Definition *Information* is data in context.

Information is data that have been processed so it is clear what they indicate. Once they are collected, data are contextualized to become information (Fig. 5.2). The context that the "50 km" refers to two points on the Interstate adds the meaning that this distance can probably be traveled (by car) in less than an hour, which can help schedule your day. In the context of a convection oven, "1000 ° F" on the display indicates that there might be something wrong with the appliance and that an intervention might be in order.

From this perspective, simply attaching units to data gives us *meaningful data*, but not yet information. The number 50 in and of itself has not much meaning, while the datum 50 km/h does. If you give that piece of data to some random person you meet in the street ("Hi! 50 km/h!"), it means something (it refers to a certain velocity), but it is not information yet. Information would be in a statement like, "I just saw a car zooming by at 50km/h!" The information here is that you inform someone about the speed of a car (or your subjective estimate thereof.)

5.3.3 Evidence: Information Compared

Information thus conceived can give rise to *evidence*, which is generally defined as "information bearing on the truth or falsity of a proposition" [196]. Evidence is information related to a conjecture or hypothesis as being supportive of it (or not). The comparison of information in support of competing conjectures helps define what counts as evidence (Fig. 5.2) and what in turn generates the knowledge that a certain overarching causal claim is true.

Evidence is generated by comparing information to reference values or standards, which prepares the information for further analysis. Actionable knowledge is usually generated from coherent evidence from multiple independent sources of information. Rules for what kind of information qualifies as evidence and how knowledge is generated are not really part of informatics but of epistemology.

Evidence should not just be treated as a list of methods that can be used to do for population health what EBM has done for clinical medicine [193]. In a very detailed and comprehensive paper, Brownson and colleagues defined evidence in the context of public health as follows:

> For a public health professional, evidence is some form of data—including epidemiologic (quantitative) data, results of program or policy evaluations, and qualitative data—for uses in making judgments or decisions" [197]

We would argue that what Brownson and colleagues call "some form of data" is in fact what we call *information*, which Mensah and Goderre define as "processed data that provides (sic) understanding" [195].

Brownson and colleagues describe three kinds of evidence that should be considered in public health contexts. They refer to (1) the causes of illness and the magnitude of risk factors, (2) the relative impact of specific interventions, and (3) how and under which contextual conditions interventions were implemented [197]. In their paper, the first kind of evidence is at the center of attention; however, causal inference also plays an important role in the other two.

If evidence is the primary basis for decision-making in population health, it can serve as the basis for evidence-based decision-making and intervention. Often, good observational (non-interventional) evidence is sufficient to start the design process for public health action. Sarah Viehbeck and colleagues recently wrote that

> in public health, the use of nonexperimental methods is often entirely appropriate and sufficient, particularly when causal chains are short and effect sizes are large [198]

In essence, we think that although interventions are part of the *post hoc* litmus test for public health knowledge, i.e., confirmation, evidence from observations is perfectly capable of supporting decisions to initiate certain public health actions.

Going back to our street encounter example above, the informational statement "I just saw a car zooming by at 50km/h" is compared to a standard: your opinion about how the observed velocity of the car compares to what you think traffic rules should allow. Just as in criminal justice, a comparison is the added ingredient that transforms information (the husband has gunpowder on his hand) into evidence (he wouldn't have if he had not fired the gun that killed his mother in law).

Definition *Evidence* is information that bears on the truth of a proposition compared to a standard

Consider a public health information system designed to aid in water-related outbreak detection, the Waterborne Disease and Outbreak Surveillance System (WBDOSS).[2] In their report on outbreaks in 2011 and 2012, Karlyn Beer and colleagues wrote about 32 drinking water–associated outbreaks that were deemed responsible for at least 431 cases of illness, 102 hospitalizations, and 14 deaths [199]. To minimize the number of false alarms, we need a definition of what constitutes a waterborne disease outbreak:

> For an event to be defined as a waterborne disease outbreak, two or more persons must be linked epidemiologically by time, location of water exposure, and case illness characteristics; and the epidemiologic evidence must implicate water as the probable source of illness [199]

According to our definition above, the information in this classification scheme becomes evidence only if it bears on the truth or falsity of the proposition that the water was the culprit. For example, what we are really interested in is whether a certain source of drinking water was, in fact, the cause of the outbreak. Only if we can find *good evidence* in support of the claim that it was can we say that we have knowledge that the cause of the outbreak was contaminated water.

5.3.4 *Knowledge from Evidence*

As discussed in Sect. 4.2.2, the traditional tripartite concept of knowledge is ascribed to Plato [163]. According to this definition, knowledge is justified, true belief. Although still in use, Gettier argued in 1963 that the tripartite definition is not

[2] https://www.cdc.gov/healthywater/surveillance/index.html.

sufficient to constitute knowledge, in essence by referring to two counterexamples in which individuals hold justified, true beliefs, that clearly do not count as knowledge [181]. Multiple strategies to defeat Gettier, e.g., counterexamples and candidates for fourth ingredients, have been suggested [200].

Despite Gettier still holding out after half a century of debate, we will refer to the tripartite definition of knowledge in the public health context. Knowledge is needed to justify the application of information at a higher level of abstraction— the result of a combination of rules, relationships, ideas, and experiences [201]. We need knowledge, which in turn should be justified by good evidence. Data become knowledge when they are transformed into information and further into *good* evidence.

For the purpose of this discussion, and without paying much attention to tomes of discussion points about what knowledge is and what it isn't, we consider information worthy of the appellation "evidence" if it can serve as the justification of beliefs that

1. turn out to be predictive in that predictions that are made based on such beliefs turn out to be correct;
2. generate hypotheses that can be tested, and
3. ideas that lead to interventions that are successful,
4. for a long time.

Beliefs qualify as knowledge, again for the purpose of this book, if they allow us to predict outcomes with satisfactory precision, if they can be translated into scenarios that allow for putting the belief to the test, and if actions based on such beliefs are consistently successful. In short,

Definition *Knowledge* is predictive, testable, consistently successful belief.

This is why *evidence*-based medicine and public health should actually be considered *knowledge*-based once the evidence has turned out to be predictive, is tested, and interventions have been designed and that are consistently successful. Of course, the decision when that point has been reached is not made by any one person, but by consensus (Fig. 5.2).[3]

Consider this information about the lead contamination of drinking water in Flint, Michigan, as summarized by David Bellinger in 2016:

> In 2014, solely as a cost-saving measure, the city began taking its water from the Flint River rather than Lake Huron. The corrosion-control treatments required by the Environmental Protection Agency's Lead and Copper Rule were, for some reason, discontinued. To make matters worse, the addition of ferric chloride to reduce the formation of trihalomethanes from organic matter increased the corrosivity of the Flint River water. The water reaching consumers was therefore 19 times as corrosive as it had been when the source was Lake Huron. The more corrosive water is, the more readily it can dissolve metals such as lead. So the lead concentration in Flint's water began to rise. In six of nine city wards, the water in 20 to 32% of the homes had a lead concentration above 15 μg per liter, a concentration that

[3] We do not have the space here to elaborate on *how* that consensus is reached. As a point of departure for such discussion, one may want to start with reading Ludwig Fleck's work on the concept of the scientific collective [202] and Miriam Solomon's discussion of the medical consensus conference process [186].

> triggers remedial action under the Lead and Copper Rule. The 90th percentile was 25 μg per liter, and in some samples the concentration exceeded 1000 μg per liter (www.FlintWaterStudy.org) [203]

Up to this point, it looks as if we receive only data and information in this quote. But the transition into evidence is hidden in the phrase "that triggers remedial action". In order to become evidence that triggers action, the information "the water in 20 to 32% of the homes had a lead concentration above 15 μg per liter" needs to be compared to allowable standards in order to become evidence that justifies action. Indeed, the Revised Guidance Manual for Selecting Lead and Copper Control Strategies prepared by the Environmental Protection Agency (EPA) has a drinking water limit for lead of 15 μg per liter.[4] Above that level, the lead concentration exceeds the *action level*, in which case water treatment has to be initiated to remedy the situation.

Accordingly, we consider it *knowledge* if a policymaker is (i) justified (by good evidence) to (ii) believe that contaminated drinking water was the cause of the outbreak (iii) if, and only if, contaminated drinking water was in fact the cause of the outbreak. In the context of knowledge, causal inference is necessary to establish knowledge about the source of the outbreak by establishing the third condition, that of truth.

Earlier we wrote that we refer to *evidence* as information that supports a specific proposition by bearing on its truth. In this sense, evidence is context-dependent, it becomes evidence by virtue of being relevant as support for a specific proposition. In public health, two kinds of propositions are at the center of attention of those who make intervention and policy decisions: more general propositions of facts (it is the case that X) and more specific propositions of causation (X causes Y).

The literature on and definitions of "all things knowledge-related" is heterogeneous. What follows is a collage of snippets picked from this literature.

In 1994, Kathryn Dean called for a new knowledge base for public health [204, 205], which she envisioned to be generated by "interdisciplinary research guided by sound theory and drawing on the range of appropriate methods" [204:218]. In artificial intelligence (AI), *knowledge-base* is defined as a set of sentences that represent assertions about the world, some of which are axioms, i.e., are not derived from other sentences [206:235].

According to Charlie Eriksson [205], new knowledge is generated in four knowledge domains that can be construed broadly as (1) population health indicators, (2) determinants of health development, (3) health impact on individuals and societies, and (4) methods for changing health determinants. The importance of causal

[4] See https://nepis.epa.gov/Exe/ZyNET.exe/P100999U.TXT?ZyActionD=ZyDocument&Client=EPA&Index=2000+Thru+2005&Docs=&Query=&Time=&EndTime=&SearchMethod=1&TocRestrict=n&Toc=&TocEntry=&QField=&QFieldYear=&QFieldMonth=&QFieldDay=&IntQFieldOp=0&ExtQFieldOp=0&XmlQuery=&File=D%3A%5Czyfiles%5CIndex%20Data%5C00thru05%5CTxt%5C00000025%5CP100999U.txt&User=ANONYMOUS&Password=anonymous&SortMethod=h%7C-&MaximumDocuments=1&FuzzyDegree=0&ImageQuality=r75g8/r75g8/x150y150g16/i425&Display=hpfr&DefSeekPage=x&SearchBack=ZyActionL&Back=ZyActionS&BackDesc=Results%20page&MaximumPages=1&ZyEntry=1&SeekPage=x&ZyPURL; page 9.

inference is directly evident in the creation of knowledge in domains 2,3, and 4, and to a certain extent perhaps even in the first.

Allan Best and colleagues discuss the definition of knowledge translation (and of other knowledge-related activities) as provided by the Canadian Institutes of Health Research (CIHR), which sees the process of "translating knowledge into improved health of the population" as "the incorporation of research knowledge into policies and practices", based on "the exchange, synthesis, and ethically-sound applications of research findings within a complex system of relationships among researchers and knowledge users" [207:321]. They view such definitions as situated in one of three categories: linear, relationship, or systems models. We will consider the systems perspective in more detail in the next section. Trishia Greenhalgh and Sietse Wieringa have recently attacked the "knowledge translation" metaphor. They think that introducing other usages of the term "knowledge" might help make the spectrum of knowledge-service situations broader and more interesting:

> [M]any non-medical disciplines such as philosophy, sociology and organization science conceptualise knowledge very differently, as being (for example) 'created', 'constructed', 'embodied', 'performed' and 'collectively negotiated' - and also as being value-laden and tending to serve the vested interests of dominant élites. We propose that applying this wider range of metaphors and models would allow us to research the link between knowledge and practice in more creative and critical ways [208].

Greenhalgh and Wieringa's point is that appreciating the multiple meanings and functions of the concept of knowledge beyond mainstream scientific knowledge, e.g., situation-specific wisdom, tacit knowledge shared by practicioners and experts, or macro-level knowledge, will enrich our perception of how to close what they call the "know-do gap".

One particularly vulnerable issue in the attempts to close that gap between science and practice appears to be lack of knowledge implementation and the reasons for and context of such lack of implementation [209] (page 152). Lawrence Green and colleagues see this phenomenon as probably due to "leaks in the pipeline", with loss of information at multiple crucial mile-markers all along the way from research funding via peer review, publication, research synthesis, the creation of guidelines, and practice.

In the biomedical sciences, Muin Khoury and colleagues recently wrote from their genomic epidemiology perspective that knowledge integration

> involves three closely related, iterative components: knowledge management, knowledge synthesis, and knowledge translation. Knowledge management is the ongoing process of obtaining, organizing, and displaying evolving evidence. [...] Knowledge synthesis is the process of conducting systematic reviews using a priori rules of evidence. [...] Knowledge translation refers to stakeholder engagement and brokering to influence policy, guidelines and recommendations, as well as the research agenda to close knowledge gaps. [210]

In 1990, Murray and Porter suggested for the public health arena that

> knowledge integration is the task of incorporating new information into a knowledge-base. This is an important and difficult task because the interactions between new information and existing knowledge can be numerous and subtle. Current knowledge-acquisition tools ignore these interactions. Knowledge integration requires an active learner following three steps: recognition, elaboration and adaptation. [211:382]

Apparently, they referred to the integration of new knowledge with existing knowledge. Green and colleagues, on the other hand, think that knowledge integration should be viewed as "the effective incorporation of knowledge into the decisions, practices and policies of organizations and systems" [207:322]. Here, knowledge integration refers to the integration of knowledge (as an intangible system of beliefs, old or new) into the public health action process.

In sum, we think that the knowledge-based approach can be an important component of causal knowledge integration. Any public health action needs to integrate input from the data-generating branches of public health (surveillance and research), information science, and philosophy. Data are transformed into knowledge by using the data ► information ► evidence ► knowledge (DIEK) process. Guidance and informatics tools for knowledge formation, translation, utilization, and integration are needed. Surveillance, epidemiology, and evaluation are major DIEK-generating areas that employ population health informatics and data science approaches and in which causal discovery and inference tools may be developed.

5.3.5 Preventive Intervention: Knowledge-Maker or Knowledge-Confirmer?

Some are apparently heavily opposed to the idea that the medical standard model for causal inference, the RCT, should serve as the basis for evidence generation in public health as well:

> To impose a narrow research model from clinical medicine (RCT) as the basis of evidence in public health would not be accepted among public health researchers and professionals […] we raise a tombstone over the RCT fanatics with the inscription: Give peace to the fanatics – but let them stay in their grave and not disturb a sound and broad evidence-based development in public health [212:242]

Another group of authors writes:

> The argument is often made that the public health evidence base is "weak" compared with other areas (medicine for example). The assumption is that a large part of this perceived weakness is attributable to the lack of studies using randomized controlled trial (RCT) designs that, when taken as a body of evidence, will enable causal inferences to be made (…) Valuable evidence about public health interventions can be gathered through RCTs, non-RCTs, and many other types of research, particularly mixed-methods approaches, depending on the question and the level of certainty required from the answer [198]

We couldn't agree more. The idea that RCTs are epistemologically superior to observational (non-interventional) studies has been cogently refuted [178, 213]. Well-designed (non-interventional) cohort and case-control studies that minimize or even eliminate the likelihood of chance and bias as an option to explain results should not be considered less valuable than (interventional) randomized trials. What is the extra ingredient that enables interventional, but not observational, evidence to generate causal knowledge? It might not be intervention per se, but preventive manipulation that provides the extra ingredient. The ability to reduce the outcome by reducing exposure is a very cogent proposal. Therefore, manipulability accounts of causation, such as Jim Woodward's [71], play a prominent role in current discussions of causal inference.

In keeping with the flow from data to knowledge depicted in Table 5.1, our DIEK model can be aligned with the general process that leads from data to knowledge in public health. Two related theoretical areas that still need to be worked out in detail so they can be tackled in practice are *data integration* and *knowledge integration*. We will address some of these issues in Chap. 7.

The integration of heterogenous data is needed for at least two purposes. First, it is needed where data that are to be queried (bottom-up) are stored in a variety of heterogeneous databases. Sujansky sees heterogeneous database integration as "the creation of a single, uniform query interface to data that are collected and stored in multiple, heterogeneous databases" [214]. For example, data integration is key in any attempt to generate knowledge from molecular research data for genomic medicine [215] by drawing on data from a multitude of publicly accessible databases that provide data at the, e.g., genomic, metabolomics, proteomic levels etc. [216]. In population health informatics, data integration is crucial for the development of surveillance systems. For example, Nsoesie and Brownstein suggest that in the context of future global influenza surveillance systems,

> the integration of data sources (e.g., the Internet and mobile phone technologies) can reduce gaps present in individual sources and systems. Data integration techniques using Bayesian ensemble and filtering methods have been shown to yield promising results both for influenza monitoring and prediction. The integration of diverse data sources or models based on a combination of different data types has the potential to improve estimates of influenza activity relative to a single system or data source. [217]

The other kind of data integration is important for the generation of computational (top-down) models that draw on different kinds of data [218]. In this case, data integration is crucial, especially when it comes to multiscale modeling [219, 220] and when paving the information highway from systems biology to systems medicine :

> The idea is not to translate ideas from one domain to another, such as translating advances in material science into improved consumer products, but to integrate data from in vitro experiments, animal models, and high- dimensional omics data with clinical data on body characteristics and function, biomarkers, and health history. [221]

5.4 Quality Transition Checkpoints

In the previous section, our focus was all about the question what constitutes good evidence that can be considered knowledge? Our response was that evidence is good if it makes good predictions, is testable, and leads to consistently successful interventions. Good evidence is *reliable* in the sense that inference based upon it leads to predictions and decisions that researchers and policy-makers are happy with for a long time. The disadvantage of this requirement is that it can only be established long after after the evidence has been evaluated.

Are there checkpoints that support the decision to promote evidence to the level of *good* before we have seen the quality of its predictions, witnessed it testability, and received the good news that interventions based on such evidence are being consistently successful? Here is a collection of candidate checkpoints that we think allows us to proceed from evidence to knowledge, moving forward. What we need to keep in mind is that we look at this question with an intervention in mind; our query is, thus, not what makes evidence so good that it is knowledge, but rather what makes evidence so good that it is useful knowledge in our population health-related context. Usefulness, in turn, is the possibility to use this evidence in ways that improve health.

Relevance First, although this should go without saying, good evidence is *relevant* to the problem at hand. Consider this quote from the abstract of a recent review in the Annual Review of Public Health:

> Legislators and their scientific beneficiaries express growing concerns that the fruits of their investment in health research are not reaching the public, policy makers, and practitioners with evidence-based practices. Practitioners and the public lament the lack of relevance and fit of evidence that reaches them and barriers to their implementation of it [209]

Basically, if evidence is irrelevant, it isn't useful. The focus on usefulness is, yet again, motivated by the goal of public health efforts to inform decision making which leads to effective action.

Robustness Second, good evidence is robust. This is what Broadbent has called the stability of a result, i.e., the characteristic of a theory or piece of evidence that it is (a) not soon contradicted by good scientific evidence, and (b) unlikely that it will soon be contradicted by good scientific evidence [80:63].

Repeatability Third, good evidence is repeatable in the sense that similar data gathering and integration efforts lead to similar evidence repeatedly: "Repeatability concerns the exact repetition of an experiment, using the same experimental apparatus, and under the same conditions" [222:5].

Reproducibility Fourth, good evidence is reproducible: "Reproducibility is … implementing the same general idea, in a similar setting, with newly created appropriate experimental apparatus" [222](page 7).

We do not have the space in this book to offer a full-fledged discussion of the topic we try to tackle here superficially. Still, we hope that our discussion will contribute to the generation of knowledge that, at some point in the future, will turn out to be useful, and perhaps even helpful.

5.5 Summary

In this chapter, we have suggested that knowledge isn't something out there for us to discover. Instead, we propose that knowledge is made. We have outlined a framework that builds on Ackoff's knowledge-hierarchy, in which data give rise to information, which leads to knowledge and finally wisdom. Our model drops the notion of wisdom, because we think it is too fraught with psychological baggage to be used in a philosophical context.

Instead, we insert the notion of evidence into the inferential sequence between information and knowledge (DIEK process). In brief, surveillance and epidemiologic studies yield observational data that are used mainly as raw material for information generation. When these data are useful in any way, they are integrated as information in models of diseases or other helpful vehicles designed to provide integrated information needed as evidence. Based on this evidence, action is justified and knowledge is generated. Knowledge conceptualized as evidence-based belief is predictive, testable, consistently successful belief, success as defined by discussion and group consensus among scientists, sometimes in collaboration with philosophers.

In the next chapter, we discuss *risk* as defined for individuals and populations. We will describe epidemiological ways of risk analysis and argue that *epidemiological risk estimation is causal explanation at the population level.*

Chapter 6
Population Risk

Abstract In the previous chapters we have focused on metaphysical and epistemological concepts of causation, in medicine and population health. In this chapter, we discuss risk estimation, the focus of public health informatics methods. First, we introduce the concepts of risk and prediction. We contrast individual and population risk and discuss why using quantitative risk estimates in individuals is problematic. We describe methods for risk estimation in population health science and conclude with the proposal that risk estimation is giving a causal explanation in population health science.

Keywords Risk · Prediction · Estimation · Causation · Explanation

6.1 Introduction

What is *risk*? In their practice-oriented discussion from the perspective of toxicology and environmental risk assessment of the use of chemicals, Malmfors and Rosing offer four definitions of *risk*: risk as (1) hazard, (2) probability of negative consequence, (3) damage that is not wanted, and (4) relative frequency of something one wants to avoid. They conclude that

> risk is, semantically speaking, a generic term, i.e., a term that denotes a family of different but vaguely interconnected concepts. All risk concepts imply that there is a possibility of damage or other unwanted consequence. They also imply a degree of uncertainty [223]

Apparently, the term *risk* has multiple meanings. Another possibility is that the above definitions describe four characteristics of the same thing. Our suggestion in this book is that – in the context of health data science - this *one thing* is a complex causation process. This view holds that the function of a constellation of risk factors is the (initial) causation process that, in turn, starts the (subsequent) pathogenetic process that culminates in clinical disease. We think that, in a sense, risk and causation are two ways to describe the same process from two perspectives. Both *risk* and *causation* refer, technically speaking, to a process moving forward in time. *Risk* is an inherently futuristic concept; the risk perspective is a prospective perspective,

O. Dammann, B. Smart, *Causation in Population Health Informatics and Data Science*, https://doi.org/10.1007/978-3-319-96307-5_6

looking forward to future adversity, while *causation* looks backward in time, from current state of health affairs back to what might have been causal events in the past.

Consider those familiar stories of great grandfathers who smoked for their entire lives and lived to see their great grandchildren getting married. How can this be, with tobacco smoking being associated with a two to fourfold increased mortality risk, even when adjusted for social status? [338] We are (of course deliberately) mixing individual and population risk here. Maybe we (inappropriately) mix the general concepts of prediction in individuals versus in populations? In what follows, we offer a few introductory thoughts about these concepts, as always from the biomedical and epidemiological angles.

6.2 Prediction

Scientific research aims at an improved understanding of the facts we want to better *understand* in order to improve our capability to *control*. This requires us to successfully predict whether a particular event will occur or not, and whether some intervention will be successful or not. Most research is therefore evaluated in a rather pragmatic way, by assessing to what extent its conclusions stand the test of time, measured as its capability to yield successful predictions.

In the health sciences, predicting the future for individuals is usually based on probabilistic population estimates. The reason why epidemiologists seek to identify risk factors of outcomes is to learn about the causal framework of such outcomes, which enables them to prevent their occurrence. Unfortunately, they often implicitly attribute causal powers to observed risk factors. This reflects the idea that causation is something out there they can detect. We, on the other hand, endorse David Savitz's view that "causal inference is just that – an inference by the interpreter of the data, not a product of the study or something that is found within the evidence generated by the study" [28].

This latter quote might be a surprise to those who strongly believe in the explanatory powers of biomedical research. Isn't this exactly what research and science are supposed to provide, i.e., proof that smoking does cause lung cancer or that drug X does cure disease Y? Alas, were it only that simple. Those who always thought this to be the case, should brace themselves for yet another quote from Savitz: "The cliché that epidemiologic studies generate only measures of association, not causation is meaningless … even experiments just generate measures of associations as well". All this boils down to the Humean idea (discussed in Chaps. 3 and 4) that causation cannot be established with certainty. Without this certainty, our predictions of health outcomes seem unjustified. Therefore, we conclude that all clinicians and health information scientists need to be disabused of the idea that absolute proof is possible outside formal logic, that clinical trials infallibly establish the efficacy of medical interventions, and that the perfect prediction of an individual's or community's future would be possible if only enough valid information were available at the necessary level of detail. We think that finding perfect predictors of your favorite health outcome is an elusive goal. Although perhaps a nice dream, it will remain a dream.

6.2.1 *Individual Risk*

For most of us, good health is more of a goal than the regular state of affairs. Many are working very hard towards that goal by trying to live the healthiest life possible, to live the happiest life possible. We exercise, we watch our diets, we don't smoke, and we focus on red wine (the one with the anti-oxidants) when celebrating the end of the work day. And yet, we all know someone who contracted the flu despite vaccination, someone who suffered a heart attack while jogging, or who was diagnosed with lung cancer although she never smoked. Even the healthiest lifestyle does not guarantee a long, healthy life. On the other hand, we also all know somebody who always drank too much, or was a lifelong smoker, but somehow managed to live to the old age of 95 and die quietly in his sleep (as one of our great-grandfathers actually did.)

So why all the effort when a good or bad longterm outcome of any lifestyle cannot be guaranteed? Why avoid all those well-documented risk factors, if you can still become sick? Why not just do whatever you please and wait for the unpredictable to occur? Yes, we'll all die sooner or later, no matter what we eat and no matter how much time we spend in the gym.

Well, the good news is that diet, exercise, and lots of sleep don't make all badness vanish, but they can *reduce your risk* of future disease and even postpone death, albeit only on average. Public health research suggests that your risk of becoming sick is lower if you eat your veggies and lead an active life, unlike those chips-munching couch potatoes. Epidemiological studies suggest that your risk of premature death is lower when you spend lots of time in your running shoes than it would be, on average, if you didn't own sneakers. But what is this really, *your risk*?

In biomedicine, the term *risk* is used in (at least) two ways. At the individual level, i.e., for a single person, being "at risk" means to have certain characteristics that are markers of the potential that this person will experience some undesirable health issue at some future point in time. Here, "risk" can be viewed as synonymous with the terms "threat" and "danger". The smoker is at risk for serious lung disease. The sloppy person jumping out of an airplane is at risk for death by faulty parachute that she didn't fold properly. The clumsy lumberjack is at risk for loss of limb. The student temping in a level 4 infectious disease research facility is at risk for infection. Individual risk thus defined can only be described at the qualitative level but cannot be quantified without taking the inferential leap from population risk to personal risk.

Personal risk is the idea that the concept of risk bears meaning for the individual. Risk is what hasn't occurred yet but could occur. And even if something has already happened to you, you can still be at risk. For example, although you had a flu-like disease last fall, you can get it again this year. Whenever you think about anything lying ahead in your life, you think about it in terms of what it will do to you, how it might affect your wellbeing, change your life. David Ropeik and George Gray have gathered information on hazards in everyday life, in the environment and in medicine. In their "practical guide for deciding what's really safe and what's really dangerous in the world around you", they define risk as "the idea that something might happen, usually something bad"[224].

This is especially true concerning personal decisions that you know will have a direct and immediate impact on your life. Who should you marry? Where should you move? Which car should you buy? Or think about health decisions: What should you eat? What preventive measures should your State Department of Public Health take? What kind of chemotherapy would be best in this particular patient's brain cancer? The way most people appear to look at risk is to use the term synonymously with *the event or occurrence to be avoided.* In this sense, *risk* is taken to be the brain cancer to be prevented, the heart attack to be avoided, the premature death not to occur.

When we look at individual risk as a personal issue, disease risk is the potential future occurrence of disease. "The ability to sense and avoid harmful environmental conditions is necessary for the survival of all living organisms" [225]. The opening sentence from Paul Slovic's seminal 1987 article on risk perception is strong motivation for thinking about risk. People look at the world out there and find that part of it is safe, while other aspects are dangerous. Our key to survival is to stay out of harm's way. In a sense, this is a quintessentially individual perspective. People like you and me, persons, view the world this way and attempt to evade potential disasters, thereby maximizing their individual benefit and optimize their future.

Three characteristics of "risk" emerge. First, risk appears to be something out there, waiting to change our life. Second, should it come, it will tend to make life worse. Third, most people will probably think about risk as being fraught with uncertainty. In short, all three characteristics can be taken together to mean *danger looming*. In keeping with these characteristics, untoward health outcomes are perceived as hazards, which can be avoided if factors that are found to contribute to the occurrence of the hazard, i.e., *risk factors*, are avoided. Thus, valid risk estimation is a prerequisite for any effort in medicine and public health that is targeted at therapeutic or preventive intervention, respectively. The risk factor concept holds that any factor identified as being associated with an adverse health outcome might be a worthwhile target for intervention. Therefore, the reliable identification of risk factors is an important research tool. Epidemiologists are charged with the identification of risk factors, and they do so by studying risk in populations, which is the topic of the next section.

6.2.2 Population Risk

Communities organize their common lives to optimize their future together. Even in situations where the outcome of the decision seems to affect individuals only remotely or after a considerable time lag, we still need to think about the potentially negative consequences of behavior and decision-making at the population level. In large groups of individuals, *risk* is estimated as the probability of new cases of said undesirable health issue (death due to parachute malfunction, loss of limb among lumberjacks, etc) over a specified period of time (incidence rate). The estimation of population risk is most commonly based on the frequentist approach to statistics and can thus be quantified.

At this point, multiple questions arise. Can we study illness risk in populations, put a number to it, and use these data to prevent illness occurrence by offering these population data to both populations and individuals? Can you use such information to predict your own future, estimate your likelihood of getting sick, and calculate your chance of dying within the next few years? As so often with technical terminology, there are multiple different concepts and definitions attached to the term *risk*. Indeed, definitions are highly context-specific. (For example, the term *stress* has very different (but related) meanings in material science and psychology.) Bankers crunch numbers and perform *risk assessments* before breaking the deal. Business decisions are governed by *risk-benefit ratios*. The influential financial consultant Glyn A. Holton starts his attempt to define risk, with a survey that ranges from subjective (Hume, de Finetti) to objective interpretations of probability (Knight) to portfolio theory. When it comes to risk measurement, however, Holton offers the rather pragmatic suggestion that it is "meaningless to ask if a risk metric captures risk. Instead, ask if it is useful" [226].

6.2.3 *Population Risk Estimates Used in Individuals*

In clinical medicine, frequentist risk estimates are used for risk description and prediction in individuals. Almost always, population data are used to communicate risk information to individual patients. The apparently naïve question posed by a patient, "What does that 10% risk mean for me, Doctor?" is a good one: it is obvious what 10% means when we refer to a population, but it is utterly unclear what 10% refers to in one individual patient. This leads to the question, what is the relationship between individual and group risk? Can we establish risk quantitatively in populations and use this information in individuals to put a handle on it and ameliorate it?

One view is that *risk* does not exist at the population level, only as a concept that applies to individuals. For example, theoretical epidemiologist Olli Miettinen holds that "risk is inherently a theoretical, nonempirical entity … (that) refers to individuals (of a given kind), whereas incidence characterizes populations" [22:249]. According to this line of thinking, risk is defined as a parameter, something beyond measurement. You can measure the baby's weight and length, and the number of days she spent in the hospital. You can also measure her blood pressure and urinary output, but you cannot *measure* her risk of, say, developing cerebral palsy or contracting the measles later in childhood. The opposite view is Rockhill's, who writes that "a risk factor is a probabilistic concept that applies to an aggregate of individuals, not to a specific individual" [227]. In Miettinen's world, the term "risk" has meaning for individuals only; it should not even be used for populations, where incidence is calculated as the likelihood of some future adverse health event over a given time span. In Rockhill's world, the term "risk" has meaning only when we are talking about populations and this (quantitative) meaning cannot be applied to individuals. The problem has been stated eloquently by Hill:

> We cannot necessarily, perhaps very rarely, pass from (the overall result of a clinical trial) to stating exactly what effect the treatment will have on a particular patient. But there is, surely, no way and no method of deciding that [32].

According to Hill and Rockhill, it is plain wrong to collect data at the population level and draw inferences with regard to individual risk based on population data.

This is standard operating procedure in medicine and public health. However, we sometimes go overboard by giving individuals numbers that correspond to percentages or probabilities, which apply only to groups of people. One solution here would be to explain to the patient that it is not the person, but the group the person belongs to that has this or that particular characteristic. The farther the individual's characteristics from the mean characteristics of the group, the less likely it is that the group probability bears meaning for the individual. The application of the probability concept in the context of individual patients ignores the fact that the *ceteris paribus* (everything else is equal) assumption is frequently violated. This is the step from probability (that a given characteristic is present) to conditional probability (that the characteristic is present given that other characteristics are present.) Modern epidemiology is based on the concept that risk can be quantified in populations and that resulting risk estimates are somewhat meaningful to individuals that are members of groups of individuals that, in turn, are similar to the populations that gave rise to the risk estimate. If at all, this makes sense only if the individual the estimate is applied to has exactly all the characteristics of the population the risk estimate comes from. This is, arguably, never the case. Thus, we believe that numbers do not have a place in conversations about health risks with individuals.

The complexity of inferences as to an individual's future based on a population's past is probably far beyond what the average patient might be able to grasp. Perception by individuals of quantitative risk information varies as widely as does the interpretation of likelihoods in general. While the chance of showers announced in the radio forecast might prompt one person to carry an umbrella all day, it might lead another not to consider this a worthwhile effort. Of course, it all depends on your definition of *chance*, which some might interpret as meaning highly likely, while others think of it as close to zero. But even in situations where the outcome of the decision seems to affect you only remotely or after a considerable time lag, or if the potential negative consequences are perceived as easily bearable, most of us still ponder the potential outcome of our behavior and decision-making. Would you travel to that remote corner of the world if the chance of acquiring the swine flu is 5%? Maybe yes. Would you jump out of the airplane if you knew there was a 5% chance the parachute might not open? Maybe not. Would you dismiss a good idea if your likelihood of being wrong is 5.1%, but not if it is 4.9%? Indeed, that is exactly what most consumers of statistical hypothesis testing results do when they use 0.05

as the *significance level* above which they feel justified to reject the null-hypothesis (of no difference between groups compared) and to accept the alternative hypothesis (of a significant difference between groups).

One reason why the point estimates of percentages, relative risks, and attributable fractions based on comparative population data have no direct implication for individuals is that the value of a point estimate and the shape of its confidence interval depend upon the background characteristics of the population they are derived from. Each individual patient necessarily differs appreciably from those that make up the group the situation-specific risk estimate is derived from, just as the individuals that make up this group differ from one another.

Although there appears to be no connection between population and individual risk, population estimates of relative risks and percentages are frequently used as information for decision making in medicine, and as information communicated by physicians to patients. Can population-based research give us a hint about individual risk at all? The question that needs to be answered is, therefore, what would the extra ingredient needed to justify the usage of population parameters as information pertinent to individuals be?

In sum, it seems plausible that applying probabilities to individuals is like comparing apples and oranges. Just as one cannot equate laboratory rats and free-ranging humans, one cannot equate the incidence of an event in populations to the risk of this event in individuals. Yes, we do it all the time, by drawing a parallel and making an inference. But sometimes, we need to be reminded that we might do this at the cost of making irrational decisions. For example, airplanes do indeed crash, albeit rarely. We all are very familiar with those nasty thoughts that linger in the back of our minds when our palms begin to sweat at takeoff. Want some numbers? When data were gathered from 3306 air line pilots, 66 crashes were documented in a total of 12.9 million flight hours. This translates into 22.3 years you have to be in the air 24/7 (current lingo for "all the time") to experience 1 crash [228]. In essence, if you fly during office hours only (8 h per day, 5 days a week) you will experience one crash in 93 years. Here is the point: Sometimes it is our anxieties and inferences that go wild, not our science.

6.2.4 Why Is All This Problematic?

It seems as if we are left stuck between a rock and a hard place with three major difficulties. First, probabilities do not apply to individuals. Second, the individual view seems to have a qualitative component that population risk does not have. Third, predictability is perceived differently by individuals and epidemiologists.

The first difficulty, that probabilities do not apply to individuals, but only to the groups they belong to, might be one reason why individuals appear to have difficulty interpreting likelihoods, or at least often misinterpret them. If this is true, why has the epidemiology-medicine collaboration, where individual decision-making based on population data has been standard operating procedure for many decades, been so successful? Perhaps because, at least in part, we tend to check the outcomes of our predictions at the population level (aggregate data), not at the individual level. Thus, the contention that individual risk does not exist might still be true, in the probabilistic sense of the term.

A few articles in the recent medical literature have dealt with this problem in various ways. Rockhill, Kawachi, and Colditz describe the problem in the context of public health versus medical applications of risk information, but they do not go deeper than stating that

> Knowledge that a factor is associated with increased risk of disease obviously does not translate into the premise that a case of disease will be prevented if a specific individual eliminates exposure (or takes a chemopreventive agent); disease pathogenesis at the individual level is a very complex process [229].

Grossi suggests moving away from probability definitions of risk towards a plausibility-based, fuzzy-logic-based definition when talking to individuals about their disease event risk [230]. Rothwell and colleagues discuss what they consider the advantages of absolute versus relative changes in risk [231]. However, all these discussions somewhat avoid the *hard question* of individual risk: How can we justify basing medical decision making and communication with individual patients on risk estimates derived from populations?

The second difficulty, that individual risk has a qualitative component not captured by probabilities, suggests that the concept of population risk quantification needs to be supplemented with a qualifier, i.e., predictability. This is qualitative, not quantitative information, based on simple experience. Some things can be predicted with high versus low accuracy (e.g., death after falling from great heights versus from a third-floor window). This is a qualitative difference, not a quantitative probability. We must ask at what point does uncertainty become certainty?

The third difficulty is that definitions of *prediction* differ. The common assumption is that we think we can predict despite our inability to predict. While epidemiologists often use the terms *association* and *prediction* synonymously, common parlance has *prediction* as *forecast*. We think that neither one is quite right in that both are too simplistic. Talk about prediction acknowledges the element of expectance of future events, the element of adversity, and the element of uncertainty. All three aspects contribute to a certain level of anxiety about the event to be predicted – alternative terms like *threat*, *hazard*, or *danger* all bear that connotation – because the event to be expected might be harmful and because its actual occurrence is uncertain.

We don't need to further explain the element of potential harm. But why the uncertainty? One reason is that illness etiology is so inherently non-deterministic in nature that any attempt at predicting (forecasting) outcomes perfectly is inherently futile. Another option would be that the etiology of illness, even if it turns out to be deterministic all the way down, is so complex that we just don't understand enough about it to come up with good predictions.

An alternative view of *risk* would entail the option to reframe risk as a complex mechanistic causal process that can be observed in individuals, but not yet predicted, until systems sciences are where they would need to be in order to fully describe a complex causal mechanistic process. Conceptualized as indicators of risk and causation, exposure and outcome are viewed as integral players in this process. In this sense, risk and causation can be viewed as two characteristics of the same thing, i.e., the process of illness development.

6.3 Population Risk Estimation

Now that we have introduced the concept of *risk in populations*, we need to take a closer look at ways how population risk is established. The most basic measures of risk in epidemiological studies are prevalence and incidence, which are percentages and rates, respectively. The prevalence of a disease is simply the number of individuals with the disease in a population at a certain point in time. Thus, it measures what percentage of a population has that disease at a certain time point. The incidence (rate) is the number of newly occurring cases of illness in a population over a defined stretch of time. Prevalence is a snapshot at a certain point in time, while incidence incorporates time in the denominator.

Measures of *relative risk* (RR) are numbers that result from the comparison of prevalence or incidence between groups that differ by one characteristic, usually a certain risk factor in *observational* (non-interventional) studies, and the intervention under study in RCTs. After a predetermined follow-up period has passed, any difference between the two groups (other than the exposure) is considered being *due to* the exposure. Measures of RR are strictly speaking not measures but estimates, because the numbers do not stand in for a tangible thing, but for a conceptual relationship between two such things, exposure and outcome. Based on these simple risk estimates, RR estimates are calculated based on data derived from samples that are sampled from underlying populations. Technically speaking, it is not the sample-based estimate that is of scientific interest, but the true, albeit unmeasurable value that quantifies the association between exposure and outcome.

A positive finding, i.e., an RR that indicates an appreciable risk increase or decrease, can be due to bias (including confounding), chance, or causation. Thus, to end up with causation by exclusion, one needs to exclude bias and chance, which is considered the case if

1. the magnitude of the RR (the effect size) is appreciable, and
2. the RR is statistically significant, and
3. bias (including confounding) has been minimized.

In Chap. 2, we already introduced biostatistics and epidemiology as important tools in causal explanation in public health data science. In this section, we outline in more detail how they are used in explanatory risk models.

6.3.1 Univariable Risk Analysis

Since the mid-twentieth century, epidemiology and biostatistics have been used jointly in *health risk estimation*. Epidemiology requires an appreciable amount of biostatistical support, and biostatistics is often applied in epidemiological contexts. Even method development in biostatistics is often motivated by newly arising analytic challenges in the health sciences.

In what follows we describe one health risk estimation method. Due to the nature of this book, this overview must remain rather brief and somewhat superficial, thus leaving much to be desired. Readers interested in a more comprehensive introduction to epidemiology and biostatistics should take a look at the excellent available textbooks, e.g., Rothman, Greenland, and Lash (2008) and Motulsky (2014), respectively. In what follows, we will use examples from the epidemiological risk studies one of us (O.D.) has published over the past two decades.

The chief approach for risk estimation is rather simple if there is just one exposure and one outcome. In 2004, we published a study conducted in a large cohort of preterm infants [232]. What follows is an abbreviated and slightly simplified version of the abstract:

> Bronchopulmonary dysplasia (BPD) and cerebral white matter damage (WMD) are neonatal disorders that occur most commonly in preterm infants. In a large multicenter database, we sought to determine whether the two disorders occur together more frequently than expected and whether BPD and other neonatal respiratory characteristics are more common among infants who develop ultrasound-defined WMD than among those who do not. In a sample of 904 infants who were born before the 30th week of gestation and survived until 36 weeks postmenstrual age, we did not find a co-occurrence of BPD and WMD above what would be expected by chance. Confounding does not seem to account for this lack of association between WMD and BPD. In conclusion, our findings do not support the hypothesis that BPD contributes to the occurrence of sonographically defined WMD.

In this study, the parents of 904 preterm newborns had agreed to let us enroll their infants as study participants. The exposure is a severe lung disorder, bronchopulmonary dysplasia (BPD), purportedly leading to the outcome brain white matter damage (WMD) that can be visualized by neonatal brain ultrasound imaging. Our goal in this study was to find out whether the two disorders are associated more strongly than would be expected by chance. This in turn is interpreted as a statistical association between the two, indicating that they might be causally related. This would be the case if the occurrence of the outcome would be statistically significantly more frequent among the exposed newborns than in the non-exposed. In what follows, we will go through the motions to demonstrate how this process works. Moreover, we will seize the opportunity to demonstrate how this process leads from data to information to evidence to knowledge, in keeping with our DIEK proposal in the previous chapter.

In order to test this hypothesis, we initially performed a very simple data analysis. First, we performed a simple cross tabulation based on the likelihood of exposure and outcome obtained from actual infants. Second, the actual co-occurrence results were then compared to the co-occurrence data one would expect to arise by chance. Third, we calculate the RR (explained below) based on the same observed occurrence data, plus a confidence interval (also explained below).

6.3.1.1 From Data to Information

In order to calculate the likelihood of co-occurrence, we simply multiply the likelihood of BPD occurrence (here 169/904 = 0.19) and WMD occurrence (46/904 = 0.05), which results in 0.19 * 0.05 = 0.0095. (Note that at this point the transition from data to information is already complete; raw numbers have obtained the status of information.) Multiplication by the number of study participants (904) gives us 9 expected cases of co-occurrence just by chance (see Table 6.1). Any number of observed cases who have both BPD and WMD that is considerably higher than 9 would be considered evidence in support of the hypothesis that the two characteristics are statistically associated.

In this initial univariable analysis, we found no appreciable difference between observed and expected numbers of infants in each group defined by the crosstabulation of WMD +/− versus BPD +/−. This is sometimes called a Null-result, and the reasoning built upon this Null result is that, as in most of all of analytical biostatistical hypothesis-testing, we have no evidence that would support rejecting the so-called Null-hypothesis, according to which BPD and WMD are not associated.

To test the hypothesis, one has to perform a rather simple calculation. In order to estimate the RR, defined as the risk for the outcome (here: WMD+) among the exposed (BPD+) relative to the risk for the outcome (WMD+) among the non-exposed (BPD). In essence, the RR equals

Definition

Relative Risk RR = (a/a + b) / (c/c + d)

According to the definition above, using the fourfold table depicted in Fig. 6.1 and the data from Table 6.1, the RR for our data would be RR = (10/46) / (159/858) = 0.217/0.185 = 1.17. This number (data) is interpreted as a risk for the outcome among the exposed (0.217) being 17% higher than the risk of the outcome among the unexposed (0.185).

Table 6.1 The co-occurrence in the entire sample (*N* = 904) of white matter damage (WMD) and bronchopulmonary dysplasia (BPD) does not appreciably exceed what would be expected if the occurrence of each were independent of the other

WMD	BPD	Observed[a]	Expected[b]
Yes	Yes	10	9
	No	36	37
No	Yes	159	160
	No	699	689

Data from Dammann et al. [232]

[a]The observed occurrence is the number of children observed in each category defined by the characteristics on the left

[b]The expected frequency is the product of the individual observed probabilities of WMD and BPD occurrence: $P(WMD \cap BPD) = P(WMD)P(BPD)$

Fig. 6.1 Fourfold table listing the possible combinations of exposure and outcome

		Outcome (Disease)		
		Yes	No	
Exposure	Yes	a	b	a + b
	No	c	d	c + d
		a + c	b + d	N

6.3.1.2 From Information to Evidence

Now that we have generated this information, it can be put to work as evidence in support of the Null-hypothesis, which states that the risk for the outcome among the exposed does *not* differ from the risk among the unexposed. Note that all analytic statistics methods are designed to test the hypothesis in Null-form, which posits that exposure and outcome are *not* associated. Information generated from observed data is used to reject that Null-hypothesis, if possible.

So much for the semantics of the testing process. The mathematical part is to calculate a *confidence interval* for the point estimate of the RR, which represents the range of values that we would expect to capture the true population value. Usually, such confidence intervals are calculated as 95% or 99% intervals, which are interpreted as saying that there is a 95% (99%) chance that the confidence interval we calculated captures the true population parameter.

Definition

The 95% Confidence Interval (CI) is the interval (C.I. lo – C.I. hi) that covers the true value of the relative risk in the population with a 95% likelihood.

The calculation of a confidence interval is simply done by taking the point estimate of the RR plus/minus a constant (1.96 for 95% intervals) times the standard error of the estimate. A more widely known and more frequently used indicator of statistical significance is the so-called *p*-value, an estimate of the likelihood that we would find a point estimate with the value we did find (or a more extreme one) in case the null-hypothesis is true. Tradition established a threshold of less than 5% ($p < 0.05$) as the conventional indicator for *statistical significance*. We always need to be aware that the *p*-value is mathematically determined by both the effect size and the sample size, i.e., the number of data-generating units in the sample used for *p*-value calculation. The *p*-value in our example for the point estimate of 1.17 happens to be 0.697, which means that we have a 69.7% likelihood of being wrong if we decide to reject the Null-hypothesis (no association between BPD and WMD) and accept the alternative hypothesis instead (association between BPD and WMD present). The large *p*-value in our example suggests that the result is not statistically significant.

Recall that the point estimate we calculated for the RR of developing WMD in case the infant *does have* BPD versus *not* was 1.17, interpreted as a 17% increase of the risk for WMD among infants *with* BPD versus infants *without* BPD. The 95% C.I. for this point estimate for the RR ranges from.67 and 2.07. In keeping with our interpretation above, we take this information as evidence in support of the notion that we are 95% certain that the interval 0.67–2.07 covers the true RR in the population of infants that gave rise to our study participants.

Of note, if the Null-value (of no association, i.e., 1.0) lies outside the 95% C.I., the result is considered significant, which correspond to a p-value <0.05. On the other hand, if the 95% C.I. includes the Null-value, the result is considered not statistically significant (as it is in our example). In general, the p-value and 95% C.I. are technically equivalent in indicating statistical significance (or the absence thereof); however, epidemiologists tend to favor the C.I., which is affected by the sample size, but not by the strength of the observed association.

6.3.2 Multivariable Risk Estimation

In the previous section we have described a univariable analysis. As the name indicates, its goal is to quantify the relationship between only one exposure and the outcome variable. In this section we discuss two important issues that arise from the recognition that univariable analysis may not suffice to establish strong enough evidence in support of a causal hypothesis. The first is *confounding*, which is the chief reason to perform a multivariable analysis. The second, related concept, is that of a *propensity score*, which is one major strategy to render causal inference from observational data achievable.

6.3.2.1 Confounding

If a risk factor and the outcome under investigation have a common cause, i.e., if a third variable influences both the risk factor and the outcome, we have a situation where a confounder, the common cause, changes the estimate of the RR that results from a univariable analysis. Let's move to another study that exemplifies this situation.

From the same study population ($N = 1506$ enrolled babies) we used for the univariable example above, we sampled 1059 infants from whom data were available for (1) the presence or absence of bacteria in the bloodstream after the first postnatal week (weeks 2–4), and (2) for the presence or absence of a severe form of retinopathy of prematurity (ROP), an abnormal vascularization of the newborn's retina that can lead to limitations of the visual field or even blindness later in childhood. The presence or absence of an abnormally prominent tortuosity of retinal blood vessels was classified as "severe" and "not severe", respectively.

Table 6.2 Late bacteremia and severe retinopathy of prematurity (plus disease)

Late bacteremia		Plus disease	
Presumed	Univariable	2.7	1.6–4.5
	Multivariable[a]	1.6	0.8–2.9
Definite	Univariable	2.5	1.6–4.0
	Multivariable[a]	1.8	1.05–2.9

Data from Tolsma et al. [233]
[a]Adjustment was made for aspirin use during pregnancy, any mycoplasmas, gestational age, birth weight z score, conventional or high-frequency ventilation on postnatal clay 28, and culture-proven tracheal infection

The main risk factor we were interested in was *bacteremia*, defined as merely clinically apparent (presumed) or microbiologically confirmed (definite). In essence, this means that in *presumed* bacteremia the presence of bacteria in the bloodstream seems highly likely to the clinician, based on the clinical appearance of the infant. However, blood cultured to retrieve direct evidence that bacteria really are present in the baby's systemic circulation does not confirm this suspicion. In *definite* bacteremia we have a similar situation, only that bacteria are found in the blood culture and can, in most cases, be classified for targeted treatment with the proper antibiotic. In Table 6.2, the two categories of the main risk factor are listed on the left displays two different RR estimates for each risk factor, univariable and multivariable. The outcome in this particular study is, as explained above, ROP with vessel tortuosity, also called *Plus disease*.

The univariable results displayed in Table 6.2 suggest that for both presumed and definite bacteremia during the second through fourth postnatal week, the risk for ROP with Plus disease is almost two - threefold increased. Both univariable results (2.7 and 2.5) are statistically significant, because their 95% C.I. excludes the Null (by definition, 1.0). The multivariable results, however, look different. First, the RR point estimates for presumed and definite bacteremia are considerably reduced from 2.7 to 1.6, and from 2.5 to 1.8, respectively. Second, only the result for definite bacteremia remains statistically significant (95% C.I., 1.05–2.9), because this interval excludes the Null (1.0). Not so for presumed bacteremia, which is associated with a 60% risk increase. However, this risk increase does not achieve statistical significance, because its 95% C.I. includes 1.0.

Now, which potential confounders were used for the multivariable adjustment? Here is the full list for ROP Plus disease we adjusted for (n.b., we also built separate models using three other definitions for severe ROP):

> Multivariable adjustments were as follows: […] aspirin use during pregnancy, any mycoplasmas, gestational age, birth weight z score, conventional or high-frequency ventilation on postnatal day 28, and culture-proven tracheal infection. [233]

All these confounders had been selected based on previous confounder analyses that established which of the variables available in our dataset were associated with both exposure and outcome, one important technical requirement for qualifying as a confounder (the other one is *not* being situated on the causal pathway between exposure and outcome, i.e., not being a *mediator* of the exposure – outcome relationship.)

6.3.2.2 Why Is This Important?

Getting our feet wet in the admittedly murky waters of epidemiological data analysis had multiple goals.

First, we wanted to clarify the role of RR point estimates in risk analyses. One should always be mindful of the effect size in light of its relative importance for populations, not just its statistical significance. While an RR of 1.1 indicates a 10% risk increase for developing flu-like symptoms over the next winter from 50% to 55%, this 10% increase might mean very little. If, however, a certain risk factor increases the risk for an untreatable kind of cancer increases from 7% to 7.7%, some might take the latter information more seriously than the former. While small effects are frequently due to confounding, as a rule of thumb, an RR <0.5 or >2.0 is often considered a potentially real effect and therefore worthy of further investigation. Moreover, the interpretation of results hinges on the definition of the comparison group, because it is the *contrast* with the control group (and how it is defined) that gives meaning to the RR by providing an answer to the question, a risk increase or decrease relative to *what*?

Second, we want you to take home the message: *never trust univariable results*. This is paramount in health data science, because all results of univariable analyses are potentially confounded, probably by more than just one confounder. This is one reason why all risk factor analyses need to be multivariable, adjusted for all potential confounders available to the health data scientist. The selection of confounder variables should not be based on univariable analyses, precisely because those can be confounded, and many of them are.

In preparation of Sect. 6.4, we need to describe one more data analysis technique that yields so-called *propensity scores*. The idea goes (roughly) like this. One runs a regression model, not with the *outcome*, but with the *exposure* as the outcome variable. This will result in a set of multiple risk factors for the exposure that all have an appreciable effect size and are statistically significant. Such models are called *most parsimonious*. They can be taken as "saturated" because no additional variable included among risk factors adds information by virtue of yielding a significant result with an interesting effect size. This parsimonious risk model for the exposure can be used to create a score that can now be used, together with the exposure variable, as a covariable in a risk model for the outcome. In essence, such models give a risk estimate that can be interpreted as the RR, with all predictors of the exposure being adjusted for. Such propensity score adjustment (another form is *propensity score matching*) makes sure that we do not attribute risk information to the exposure variable that should, in fact, be attributed to the joint effect of factors that led to the exposure.

This kind of situation occurs especially in one kind of analysis that is of crucial importance for the argument we will now make. This special situation occurs in observational studies (not in Randomized Clinical Trials), where the goal is to calculate the risk reduction associated with an intervention, such as a certain drug. Here, we need to be sure that we do not attribute the risk reduction (or increase) to the drug, but to the host of reasons that led to the prescription of the drug, such as special indications or other factors contributing to the decision to prescribe it. The concept is called *confounding by indication* and can be addressed by proper consideration and usage of propensity scores.

We can now turn our attention to the first part of our argument in this chapter, the idea that *risk assessment is causal explanation* of why the outcome occurred more frequently among the exposed individuals compared to their non-exposed peers.

6.4 Risk Estimation as Causal Explanation

In the previous section we have described the risk estimation process, albeit only very superficially. In this section, we suggest that in health data science the causal explanation process and the risk estimation process are the same. We think that it is important to bring and discuss the two issues together. The argument is rather simple. If we want to explore what constellation of risk factors explains illness occurrence, we need to extract them from the collected data, put them in context, and find out how they relate to one another. This resembles very much what is called a *causal explanation.*

Health data science is about generating useful information from health data in order to gather evidence that justifies knowledge *for action*. Thus, it is paramount to ensure that health data science results can be used as evidence, and that the knowledge generated in this way can justify the intervention. The effective modification of a health care or prevention process asks for a causal explanation of such process. Again, to identify risk factors and to put them in relation to one another is to propose *a causal explanation* for such process.

Consider the following statements:

1. The outbreak occurred because the bug was in the mayonnaise.
2. We must change our strategy because health care cost continues to increase.
3. Maternal mortality decreased because of the implementation of an effective handwashing policy.

All these statements include an explanatory part (X is/was the case *because* Y is/was the case). Statement 1 explains a food poisoning epidemic by pointing to the source of the infection (bug in mayonnaise) which is considered the most likely cause of the outbreak. Statement 2 refers to rising cost as a motivation for action, and as justification for a change in the modus operandi. Statement 3 attributes the success of an intervention to a previously instated intervention. The reason for all these causal explanations is not just to satisfy our curiosity, but to generate knowledge that can be used in the future to deal with similar situations. The assumption is that proper causal interpretation of risk factors helps identify tools and targets for intervention design. From this perspective, analytical epidemiology is all we need to do, and arguably all we can do. Note that preventive intervention can do without knowledge about the biological process that leads from risk factor or intervention to outcome. In neither the mayonnaise nor the handwashing example above is knowledge about the underlying microbiological mediator (the bug) necessary for successful intervention; not eating the burger and frequent handwashing will do the job, respectively.

6.4.1 Risk Factors and Causes

We have seen that epidemiologists search for causes of illness. They do this by identifying risk factors for diseases, thereby providing causal explanations. The basic epidemiological research tools used to gather evidence in support of hypotheses about health risk factors, and thereby of causal claims in the health sciences are study design and data analysis.

As outlined above, such analyses can be done by gathering large groups of individuals who have a certain risk factor. This risk information is then contrasted with risk information from an appropriate comparison group of individuals without the risk factor. The resulting RR is considered indicative of a risk factor if it is plausible, free of bias, unlikely to be a chance observation, repeatable in various populations and study scenarios, leads to successful predictions, etc. Acceptable risk factors, in turn, are considered causal, and are used as targets for disease centered interventions in medicine and for prevention-centered intervention in public health.

Thus, the following questions arise. When do we know that a certain risk factor for a disease is indeed a cause of a certain disease? In other words, at what point does risk information become causal information? What kind of evidence is needed to justify this leap? Can risk factors be acted upon in biomedicine and public health before evidence for causation is gathered and sanctioned by the biomedical community? In fact, the underlying more fundamental question is, what is the relationship between the concepts of disease risk and disease causation, and between risk factors and causes? We will also speculate as to what consequences our explication of that relationship might have for the metaphysical and epistemological discourse of risk and causation in medicine and public health.

Risk factors are established by means of estimates of RR derived from simple calculations based on data from populations. Technically, these are statistical *correlations*, although statisticians will not let you get away with it. We are using the term correlation as synonymous with *association*, which usually makes statisticians cringe. At the most superficial level, experts in epidemiology and biostatistics follow the standard notion, “correlation is not causation” [234]. The assumption is that one cannot interpret an observed statistical correlation (association) between two variables as causal without further ado. Multiple options are available when facing this dilemma. First, one can subscribe to the idea that the right sort of scientific data operation can transform information based on statistical associations and can somehow infuse measures of RR with causal meaning. Second, one may take the soft mystical stance, which holds that RRs are just superficial, indirect indicators of a causal association, which in and of itself cannot be observed. The third is the hard mystical (Humean) stance, which denies the existence of causation as feature of nature. Fourth, we have a somewhat provocative version of the first option above, which is the view that risk factors and causes are two perspectives on the same thing, called *etiology* of illness (as outlined in Chap. 3). A fifth and even more provocative claim would be to hold that risk factors for, and causes of illness *are the same thing*.

The technical way to arrive at causation in the health science is by conducting randomized controlled trials (RCTs). In the next section, we elaborate on this topic with particular emphasis on the notion of epistemological superiority of randomized controlled intervention studies (randomized clinical trials) over observational non-interventional studies.

6.4.2 Randomized-Controlled Trials as Cause-Makers

Some physicians and biomedical researchers think of RCTs as causation-makers. For example, Kovesdy and Kalantar-Zadeh[1] refer to the "association is not causation" paradigm with reference to the presumed causation-making of RCTs when they write that "a frequent lament in Nephrology is the lack of randomized controlled trials (RCTs), and thus the inability to conclusively establish a cause-and-effect relationship between an exposure and an outcome" [235].

The epistemological weight of the RR is considered maximized by the RCT's capability to achieve all three of the following criteria:

1. the effect size to be detected is pre-conceived;
2. the sample size is calculated *pre hoc* for the effect size to be statistically significant; and
3. the randomization scheme and blinding minimize bias and confounding.

We'd like to consider the possibility that not only randomization raises the epistemological value of results from RCTs, but that intervention also contributes to such increase. Indeed, the two concepts are closely related. Intervention studies without randomization, or non-randomized controlled studies, are feasible and can deliver useful results. However, randomization is rarely, if ever, performed without subsequent intervention. Thus, in the present context, the contrast of interest might

[1] We are using this quote merely as an illustration how the purported epistemic value of RCTs as causation-makers is taken for granted in the medical research community. The quoted sentence is the first in Kovesdy and Kalantar-Zadeh's introduction; the remainder of their paper is a very thoughtful discussion including "a description of the various pros and cons of RCTs and of observational studies (and the argument) that it is simplistic to rank them solely based on pre-conceived notions about the superiority of one over the other" [235]. See also [236].

not be so much the one between intervention and observation (in the sense of non-intervention), but the one between randomization versus non-randomization.

What is it about randomization that admits of justified causal inferences? In a simple randomization scheme employed in the setting of an RCT, a large number of study volunteers is allocated to one of (at least) two groups. In the medical context, these two groups are frequently an intervention arm and a control arm in which a potential therapeutic and a placebo or different therapeutic are administered to the volunteers, respectively. The outcome of interest, e.g., improved health or prolonged survival, is ascertained in identical ways in both groups. The idea is that if all these components of the RCT are implemented according to the rule-book, a difference in the outcome between the groups can be causally attributed to what defines the contrast between them. Any systematic or chance difference between the two groups invalidates the underlying causal assumption.

The background situation is as follows. If the allocation process is truly random and unbiased, the law of large numbers (J. Bernoulli, 1700–1782) holds that the two groups will become on average more alike the larger the number of individuals grows in each group. Since this similarity holds true for all characteristics of the groups, known and unknown, the randomization process decreases the likelihood that third variables confound the relationship between exposure and outcome. In other words, if a large enough number (e.g., more than a few hundred) of volunteers is randomized into two groups, the two groups will exhibit the same average age, height, weight and so forth. They will also have the same average unmeasured, unidentified, and unknown characteristics. Therefore, in an RCT, the group exposed to an intervention should differ from the group not exposed to it by no other characteristic but the exposure. Therefore, the argument goes, any outcome difference between the groups is likely to be caused by the exposure. While this may well be the case, the conclusion is not watertight, because one simply cannot exclude the possibility that an unmeasured causal factor is distributed unequally between the two groups by chance despite randomization. But if it is not the randomization scheme that infuses causation into RCTs, what else makes members of the biomedical community so certain about this?

One possible answer is that the quality of the RCT that justifies causal inferences, usually attributed to the exposure allocation by randomization, might better be attributed to the exposure administration by intervention? All randomized studies come with an intervention in tow. In such cases, we cannot tell whether the randomization or the intervention determines the causal inference. However, some intervention studies come without randomization, for example in observational cohort studies where exposures are allocated by study participants themselves, not by researchers. Other studies are randomized, but not blinded. Blinding, and particularly double-blinding, is supposed to reduce, or even eliminate, confounding. Intervention, however has one additional evidence-generating advantage: interventions interfere with illness etiology, so that the intervention effect can be predicted based on current biological and sociological knowledge, which raises the epistemological value of intervention studies.

6.5 Summary

In this chapter, we have discussed the concept of risk, and what it means for individuals and populations. Although risk estimates from populations are generally used in communications about risk with individuals, our discussion appears to support the general notions that personal and population risk are two very different things. We have also worked out that causes and risk factors are two characteristics of the same thing, the etiology of illness. Finally, we have outlined how risk estimation works in epidemiology and biostatistics, and we propose that risk estimation is giving a causal explanation in population health science.

Chapter 7
Integrating Evidence

Abstract In this concluding chapter we describe our view how different kinds of information are integrated in order to arrive at causal explanation in population health science. In particular, such information comes from individuals and populations (target), from epidemiology and the bench sciences (method), and from observation and experiment (manipulation). We discuss recent "systems" approaches in biology, medicine, and epidemiology in the section on "method" and the question what it is about "manipulation" that convinces many of its capability to support causal inference. In the final section, we look at complexity versus simplicity and suggest that the simplification inherent in epidemiological evidence generation may be an asset, not a liability.

Keywords Information · Evidence · Integration · Systems biology
Systems medicine · Systems epidemiology · Complexity

7.1 Introduction

Those who work in different sectors of health care and public health rely on different *knowledge models* of illness causation, health outcomes, and intervention effectiveness. At least three perspectives can be distinguished that shape knowledge about health and illness.

First, the *target-oriented perspective* pays primary attention to the individual patient or to entire populations. Second, the *manipulationist* perspective contrasts experimental with purely observational results. Third, the research *methodology*-oriented perspective draws either on results from basic laboratory science or from epidemiologic studies in humans.

Different combinations of knowledge models are employed for different purposes, depending on the task at hand. For example, nurses and medical doctors tend to take the individual patient perspective and rely heavily on experimental data from both basic science and clinical epidemiology (RCTs). They ask: Might this exposure have contributed to this patient's disease? Will this drug improve her outcome? Their first-hand experience in clinical care usually represents a large component of

O. Dammann, B. Smart, *Causation in Population Health Informatics and Data Science*, https://doi.org/10.1007/978-3-319-96307-5_7

their clinical knowledge. Epidemiologists and public health researchers are obviously more likely to take the population perspective. Might this or that exposure contribute to disease occurrence in populations in general? Will this drug or community intervention improve health in this and other populations? Their knowledge is rooted in data obtained from populations, perhaps with a focus on observational epidemiological studies. Geneticists take either the individual or population perspective, but rely mainly on experimental basic research or observations in individual patients and/or groups of patients.

How can these multiple knowledge models be integrated into a common model that will help us improve our understanding of causation processes and intervention effectiveness, such that we can take advantage of that knowledge to improve health?

In this chapter, we propose the concept of *evidence integration* for public health informatics.[1]

7.1.1 Evidence in Public Health

In 2000, Charli Eriksson published a review in the Scandinavian Journal of Public Health entitled *Learning and knowledge-production for public health: a review of approaches to evidence-based public health* [205]. Eriksson suggests that evidence-based public health needs to integrate knowledge from the domains of health *distribution, determinants, consequences, and interventions.* He takes cardiovascular health as an example of successful public health activities and offers a schema that distinguishes four generations of methodological approach to the problem. Beginning in the 1950s and 60s, the clinical generation of prevention approaches came from clinical medicine and focused on single risk factors. The subsequent bioepidemiological generation embraced the multiple cause paradigm and prevention became its goal. Socioepidemiological work for public health action and subsequent environment and policy-oriented work for health promotion entered the scene more recently. Eriksson points out that the knowledge base of each of these generations of prevention research and intervention was different, coming from medical knowledge, then integrating progressively broader sociological theories. We have currently reached the stage of integration of systems theory, which we will expand upon in the next section.

[1] We prefer using the term *evidence integration* to the more common *knowledge integration* and *information integration*. Knowledge integration has been defined as "the process of synthesizing multiple knowledge models (or representations) into a common model (representation). Compared to information integration, […], knowledge integration focuses more on synthesizing the understanding of a given subject from different perspectives." (Wikipedia, accessed 6/19/2012). In keeping with our DIEK-model (see Sect. 6.3), this chapter is about evidence, not so much about information or knowledge.

Eriksson further summarizes evaluation strategies for each generation and an outcome model for public health, based on a report published by the European Commission Directorate at around the same time [237]. He concludes that

> Public health actions need grounding in political decisions and in ethical considerations. This also requires that the actions be based on scientific knowledge and practical experiences. Therefore, public health workers need epidemiological knowledge for making priorities and evidence-based methods for public health actions.

Although Eriksson is apparently no fan of mincing words (he quotes Paula Braveman when he states that we should "join forces against inequalities and poverty instead of splitting hairs" [238] – and we fully agree!), the way in which he puts knowledge in relationship to evidence is interesting. Apparently, he sees knowledge bases (plural) as providers of *evidence*. Our DIEK model (see Chap. 5) is a little more simplistic in that regard; perhaps, we should modify our DIEK model by inserting a feed-back option between knowledge and the DIE sequence (Fig. 7.1), which can also include the actions that are justified by inferences and explanations that come from DIE and/or the knowledge it generates. In this context, *action* refers to intervention of any kind, be it laboratory research, epidemiological intervention studies, or new health policies.

Data turn into information the moment they are collected. When we apply a household survey in a certain region, the data become information the moment the pencil hits the paper, because the numbers are put into context, simply by being answers to specific questions that provide the context. We put specific questions into that survey to organize our thought system about the topic at hand, e.g., population census in a region in a particular year. Now that we have these data in hand in the form of workable information, we can generate hypotheses to test, for example, hypotheses about the relation between variables, about predictors of health and illness, about the prevalence of risk factors and health outcomes in certain areas, and so forth.

In previous chapters, we have outlined that causal explanation and reasoning is a crucial part of *all* decision-making in public health and, therefore, in public health data science and informatics. In this chapter, we suggest that the integration of evidence from the target, manipulation, and methodology perspectives may help to make headway in causal inference and explanation (Fig. 7.2). In the next sections,

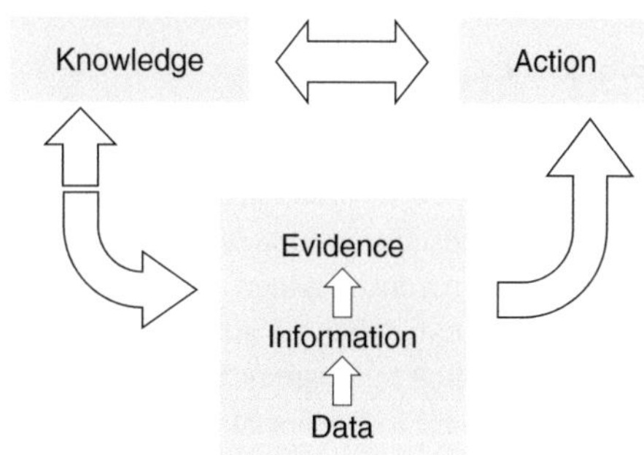

Fig. 7.1 Feedback between knowledge and action, and the DIE sequence

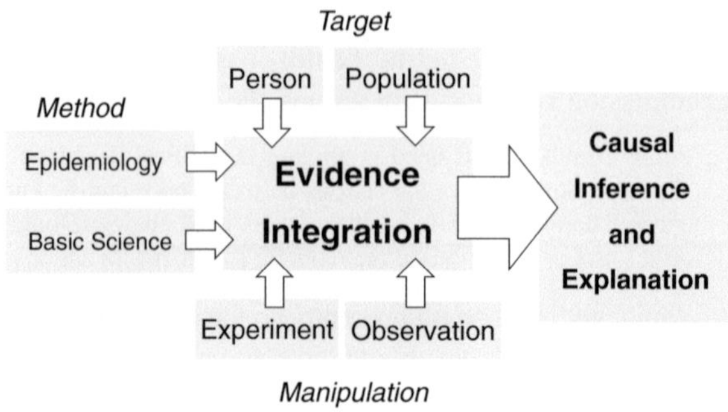

Fig. 7.2 Evidence integration accommodates considerations from target, method, and manipulation as prerequisites for causal inference and explanation

we briefly describe how this project is currently tackled and how we think it could be expanded towards better causal inference and explanation.

7.2 Target

We have already addressed the target perspective in the sections on individual and population risk in Chap. 6. We encourage our readers to refer back to those sections and return here.

7.3 Method

Illness is the result of a variety of antecedents and circumstances. Infectious diseases, congenital disorders, birth defects, traffic injuries, and socially induced health inequity are affected by social, biological, and psychological risk factors. As heterogenous as these exposures and outcomes are, the research methods applied to explore their relationships differ substantially. It is not surprising that the *method* perspective is at the center of attention of medical and public health research.

7.3.1 Systems Health

The current frameworks that cover multi-methodological evidence integration in the health sciences are *systems biology* [239–242] and *systems medicine* [221, 243–245]. Some have recently added *systems epidemiology* into the mix [142, 246–249]. Perhaps one can subsume all three under the term *systems health sciences.* All three bear importance for systems health at the population level. In order to define systems health, we need to further clarify multiple concepts in medicine, epidemiology, and philosophy of science, from the systems perspective. What might *systems health* look like and what is needed to get there?

The idea is to envision and design research programs dedicated to health improvement via truly interdisciplinary approaches that appreciate the whole spectrum of human health at all bio-psycho-social levels. Such approach has been proposed and discussed in the past [250–252], but only now do we begin to have the computational and institutional resources to bring such ideas towards application. A close collaboration between health, computer, and data scientists (as well as the law and the humanities) is needed to pull this off. In what follows, we outline a strategy for achieving this goal by building on concepts from systems biology, epidemiology, medicine, and population health.

We see systems health as the ideal outcome (*goal, end, telos*) of systems medicine and public health, which in turn relies on the generation of applicable information from both systems biology and systems epidemiology. Systems approaches are distinct from other approaches to research (here: biology and epidemiology) and practice (here: medicine and public health) in two major ways.

First, a systems perspective provides the proper canvas for data collection and design of networks means for data analysis. The idea of a systems perspective, in turn, is rooted in the concept called systems theory, originally called *general system theory* [253] by Ludwig von Bertalanffy (1901–1972). In this theory, observed phenomena are not perceived in isolation, but as interacting parts of systems. These systems, in turn, are conveniently defined by the researcher and her team, who might be interested in molecular systems at the level of the cell, or in metabolic systems at the level of the person, or in inter-personal systems at the level of a family. The main issue is not to observe characteristics of individual parts isolated within a system to understand the particular role of the part of the system, but to learn about the joint function of multiple parts working together to understand the behavior of the whole system. In essence, systems scientists see the forest first, then focus on the trees. The important theoretical parallel that comes to mind here is that of a mechanism, which has always played an important role implicitly in biomedical research, but has recently become an explicit focus of interest for philosophers of science [73, 254, 255].

Second, research at the systems level employs a computer-based infrastructure for the biostatistical analysis of increasingly large datasets that capture data about many parts of a system. It also uses information about parts or even the whole system for computer-based simulation of the workings of the system under investigation. Modeling is an integral part of systems biology, of systems epidemiology, and of systems medicine. Computational modeling has been part of the sciences for a long time and has made invaluable contributions to our understanding of the dynamics of processes as complex as the weather and life down to comparatively simple mechanisms in physics and chemistry. Since understanding is the goal, we subscribe to the view that modeling is a way of thinking that brings us beyond predictions towards explanations and the illumination of uncertainties [218, 256].

7.3.2 Systems Biology

Over the past years, a broad research endeavor has been initiated under the name systems biology [239–242]. The major thrust of this field is the elucidation of biological mechanisms at the systems level, using a combination of computational and experimental approaches. Although not enshrined in the term, the word *systems* – at least in the systems biology context – is often restricted to molecular systems at the sub-cellular level. The main approach of systems biologists, narrowly defined, is to move from experimental studies to computational models, and back, each time improving the experiment/model by integrating information from the other side. The major goal of systems biology is to improve, accelerate, and advance our understanding of cellular mechanisms by tapping into the full repertoire of basic research techniques and modern computer science.

If epidemiological and biostatistical techniques are traditionally rather computer-intensive methodologies, this applies even more to the related and overlapping fields of bioinformatics [257] and computational systems biology [241]. Both fields have something unique to offer for potential integration with epidemiology. Indeed, "molecular epidemiology … is rapidly moving from evaluation of single candidate genes, one at a time, to consideration of entire pathways … Still, most reports are limited to relative risk estimates from each factor considered one at a time or in pairwise combinations, using very traditional epidemiologic analysis tools" [258]. It is exactly this lack of new analytic tools that needs to be tackled if biological pathway analysis is to be included within epidemiological thinking.

Bioinformatics is an "area of science that uses computational approaches to answer biological questions" [259]. Part of the bioinformatics methodology offers tools to analyze large data sets (e.g., from microarrays). However, much of the statistical methodology is based on the concept of data reduction [260]. In essence, cluster and factor analytic approaches reduce the information from many data points into clusters or factors that are then treated as single variables. Indeed, "many of these techniques will be familiar tools (for the experienced biostatistician) called by a new label or applying a new jargon" [261].

More than a decade ago, Kitano suggested taking a system level approach in performing biological research:

> Molecular biology has uncovered a multitude of biological facts, such as genome sequences and protein properties, but this alone is not sufficient for interpreting biological systems. Cells, tissues, organs, organisms and ecological webs are systems of components whose specific interactions have been defined by evolution; thus a system-level understanding should be the prime goal of biology. Although advances in accurate, quantitative experimental approaches will doubtless continue, insights into the functioning of biological systems will not result from purely intuitive assaults. This is because of the intrinsic complexity of biological systems. A combination of experimental and computational approaches is expected to resolve this problem. [241]

This concept has been implemented on the cellular level, with biochemical receptor signalling pathways [262–264] and the heart [265]. More recently, suggestions have been published to bring systems biology to the bedside under the name systems medicine [221, 243–245].

7.3.3 Systems Medicine

The call for application of this concept towards better medical diagnosis and intervention has become audible, suggesting to move from systems biology towards systems medicine [221, 244, 266–268].

Systems medicine "incorporates the complex biochemical, physiological, and environmental interactions that sustain living organisms" and "exemplifies the connectivity and integration at multiple levels [...], expanding medicine beyond reductionism" [266]. It is "the interdisciplinary approach wherein physicians and clinical investigators team up with experts from biology, biostatistics, informatics, mathematics and computational modelling to develop methods to use new and stored data to the benefit of the patient" [268]. In essence, systems medicine is the incorporation of patient background and clinical information with omics-based biological data into computer-based decision support systems. One recent twist to the developing story of systems medicine uses the name "P4 medicine" [245, 269]. Here, the idea is to make systems medicine not only comparable to what has been called personalized [270, 271] or individualized medicine [272], but also predictive, preventive, and participatory [245], three concepts well-known to population health scientists.

In 2003, Collins, Green, Guttmacher, and Guyer published "a blueprint for the genomic era" prepared by the US National Human Genome Research Institute [273]. They offer their views on how to establish "robust paths from genomic information to improved human health" and discuss "grand challenges" met by scientists in all fields that contribute to three genome-related areas in which Collins and colleagues envision genomic science to improve the status quo: biology, health, and society. The authors also discuss six cross-cutting elements, one of them being computational biology, and predict that "all future biomedical research will integrate computational and experimental components." More than a decade later, their prediction has turned out partially correct, partially incorrect, in an interesting way; correct in that what they call *computational biology* has gained traction as *systems biology*, and incorrect in that one important research area has not yet fully participated in these developments, i.e., population health science.

7.3.4 Systems Epidemiology

The goals of systems medicine can be achieved by complementing systems biology techniques with systems epidemiology strategies. We believe that inferences for diagnosis, treatment, and prediction in groups of patients should not be based solely on data generated in bench experiments and computational models of these. Instead, integration is needed of data from simple systems experiments with data from population-based studies, each one supplemented with in silico simulations. Together with improved interdisciplinary discourse, such strategy will contribute to a better systems medicine (Fig. 7.3), by generating a deeper and broader

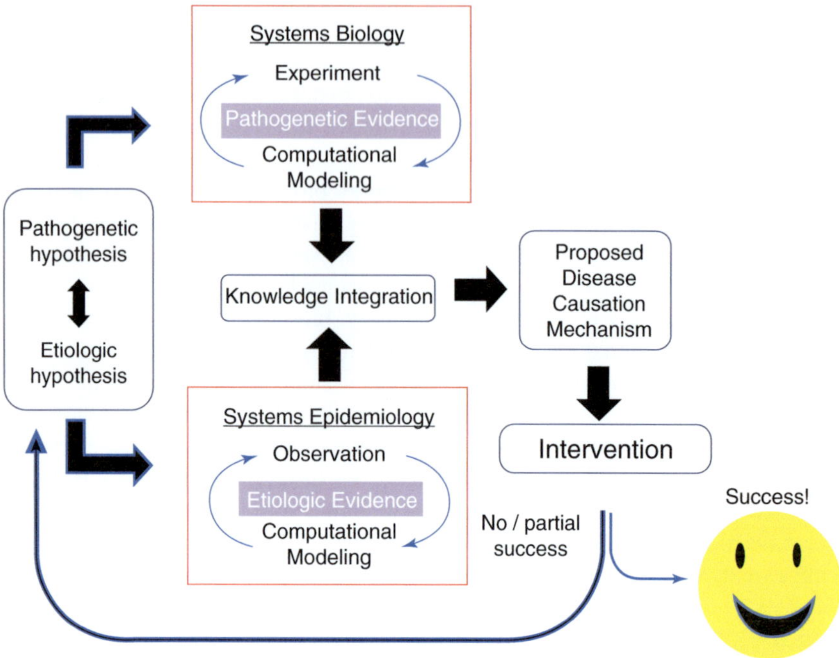

Fig. 7.3 Systems epidemiology and systems biology as a two-pronged approach require the integration of knowledge that results from both. (Reprinted with permission from Dammann et al. [142].)

understanding of biological and pathogenetic mechanisms at multiple levels, from cell to human populations [142].

In 1993, Dean Emeritus of the Harvard School of Public Health, Julio Frenk, used the term *bioepidemiology* as a name for "the study of the biological determinants, risk factors, and consequences of health processes in populations, as well as the use of methods and techniques derived from the biological sciences to characterize such phenomena" [274]. Others at that time called this idea "molecular" [275, 276] and "biomarker epidemiology" [277]. Other terms that denote the same or closely related fields are genetic [25], genomic [278, 279], and epigenetic epidemiology [280]. One key issue similar to all these approaches is the measurement of biochemical markers (or "biomarkers") in individuals with the goal to assess the role of such markers in disease and health processes. Another is, again, that all rely heavily on computational analyses.

The "rapprochement between genetics and epidemiology" [25] dates back to the concept of population genetics. Over the past decades, the overlapping disciplines of genetic [25] and molecular epidemiology [24] have been developed to bring both approaches closer together, culminating in *human genome epidemiology* [26, 279]. The major type of epidemiologic study in this field, i.e., genome wide association studies (GWAS) [281], has received lots of attention, but also generated criticism and calls for caution [282].

Now that the human genome is published [283, 284], the relatively young discipline of "genomics" [285] has developed into the "structural and functional studies of genomes" [286]. One of the major driving forces is the increasing use of microarray technologies [287], with whole human genome microarrays [288] being implemented in etiology research. Additional "omic" advances at the protein [289], peptide [290], transcript [291], and metabolite [292] levels will soon be integrated. For example, one recent proposal suggests a five-step approach that involves the selection of appropriate genetic networks, their reconstruction using gene expression data, the identification of differentially regulated genetic networks by comparison of normal and abnormal systems, and subsequent perturbation experiments and traditional association studies [293].

While genome epidemiology and GWAS studies propose to widen the search for genetic risk factors for human disease, others have suggested deepening the search. From her cancer epidemiologic perspective Cornelia Ulrich and colleagues wrote in 2006 that "mathematical modeling will allow us to link epidemiology to systems biology and will help drive our understanding of cancer etiology and cancer biology" [294]. Along the same lines, Eiliv Lund and Vanessa Dumeaux have proposed "a new research discipline, systems epidemiology, that seeks to integrate pathways analyses into observational study designs to improve the understanding of biological processes in the human organism" [249].

Molecular biologists perform experimental pathogenetic studies in the laboratory. This work relies heavily on the use of animals and simpler systems. The obvious advantages are lower costs and faster turnaround, with downsides being difficulties of extrapolation to the human system and the limitations associated with only one or a few independent variables that can be modified in order to observe changes in the dependent variables. One way to respond to Frenk's suggestion would be to use molecular biology methods to generate data for epidemiologic studies. One example for this view is Nicholson's suggestion to use comprehensive phenotyping in molecular epidemiology research [295]. In this approach, *global systems biology* information is used in the epidemiologic setting. Another example is *environmental systems biology* [296], a methodological paradigm proposed for what has been called *enviromics* [297], which Toscano and Oehlke read "to mean interactions of the complete environment, or *envirome*, with human genomes" (italics in original) [296].

A second way to interpret Frenk comes close to what cancer epidemiologist Cornelia Ulrich and co-authors [294] envision as the three benefits for epidemiologists from systems biology: helping predict biologically relevant system outputs, being quick and inexpensive, and the potential to incorporate biological pathways into statistical analyses (the latter point is probably identical to the concept illustrated in the previous paragraph). However, this proposal does not go beyond suggesting links between epidemiology and systems biology. In what follows, we suggest melting the two approaches into one. Moreover, we suggest to let the term *systems* be rather inclusive, not only on the molecular level, but also to include other systems, at the individual and inter-individual (social) levels.

In a third interpretation of Frenk's suggestion, epidemiologic observations in human populations and biological in-vivo, in-vitro, and in-silico modelling would be integrated. In-silico observations in modelled populations would then supplement epidemiology and biology in their contributing to one comprehensive framework for disease causation research. Such an approach, supplemented with computational population modeling is how we envision systems epidemiology to go beyond current epidemiologic approaches by moving from the observation of associations between exposures (risk factors) and health outcomes towards the observation of disease occurrence processes in individuals at the group level.

Risk factor identification should be tackled using systems medicine approaches, which call for the integration of molecular, genetic, demographic, health history data at the individual level [245]. If such individual data would then be explored in datasets that include many individuals, disease patterns could be compared between individuals and populations using the same information and variables. This would be an expansion of the *network of networks* approach [245], directly comparing the process of disease causation (pathogenesis) in individuals with the risk-to-illness process (etiology) in populations.

Using this framework, systems epidemiology might be able to help us accept or reject the notion that "forecasting in individual cases remains out of reach" [298:93]. If completely successful, such program might even help us determine, at the deepest possible level of analysis, whether disease causation and risk mechanisms are deterministic (and complexity prevents us from accurate prediction [298:93]), or whether accurate prediction of health outcomes will remain an elusive goal, at least until we find smarter ways of data generation, analysis, and inference.

Investigators have begun to model in-silico clinical trials [299] and now call biology-based approaches in the etiology of complex genetic disorders [300]. This is what systems epidemiology could deliver. While the epidemiologic subdisciplines enable scientists to include molecular data in traditional epidemiological data analysis, "systems epidemiology" includes computational simulation usually not included in epidemiology. In essence, a unique research methodology needs to be developed that enables disease etiology researchers not only to measure molecular markers in humans and associate/correlate these with disease risk, but also allows for the implementation of such knowledge in subsequent virtual molecular biologic experiments in the human system. Such an approach would ensure a common conceptual framework for both observation and experiment.

Moreover, fascinating approaches could be developed in research areas with ethical constraints such as cognitive neuroscience and developmental biology. Although this suggestion might sound vague and utopian, we suggest (and hope) that the future might hold such an approach in stock. Indeed, the future might have already begun, since "even whole-patient models for specific disease, such as obesity and diabetes, are being developed for prediction of disease development and drug discovery" [241].

We'd like to make two additions to Collins, Green, Guttmacher, and Guyer's 2003 prediction that "all future biomedical research will integrate computational and experimental components" [273].

First, epidemiologic research will play a crucial role in future biomedicine. Epidemiologists not only map disease frequency and distribution in populations, but as we demonstrated in Chap. 5, also help generate knowledge about the etiology and prognosis of illness by conducting observational studies and test treatments in randomized trials. Much of the progress in medicine and public health would have been impossible without the work of epidemiologists. Modern epidemiologists also embrace biology, as documented by successes of more recently developed epidemiologic disciplines such as biomarker epidemiology [301], molecular epidemiology [302], genetic epidemiology [303], epigenetic epidemiology [280], and human genome epidemiology [26], which evolve rapidly and will contribute the better health in the years to come [304]. However, most important for our suggestion is that computational modeling has become an integral part of epidemiologic research, supplementing risk factor epidemiologic studies in a rather interesting way.

Second, we predict that computational platforms will offer the tools to bring the worlds of epidemiology and lab experiment closer together. More specifically, systems epidemiology data combined with results from systems biology projects will yield disease occurrence models that cover both pathogenetic and etiologic aspects of disease development, treatment, and prognosis (Fig. 7.3).

7.4 Manipulation

Health-related hypotheses are usually tested by way of designing observational or intervention studies (see Chap. 2 for a description of this process). Evidence from intervention studies such as randomized trials is obviously considered particularly important for population health action. In one of the most recent books on population health informatics, the author of the chapter on inferential and descriptive statistics states that "the only way to prove causation is through experiment" [2:149]. If he were right, smoking would still not cause lung cancer.

From the public health informatics perspective, we are most interested in approaches that help us assess evidence from randomized trials. As an example, let us take a closer look at one of the available software systems for decision making in the health sector, GRADE.[2]

The system was developed by the GRADE Working Group, who entered the scene at around 2003 with a paper in the Canadian Journal of Medicine. The abstract stated that they

> were unable to identify health care research that addressed, either directly or indirectly, the best way to present grades of evidence and recommendations (in health care) [305]

In that particular paper, the authors discussed the use of symbols like numbers, letters etc. in grading systems. At that point, they were in the process of developing

[2] https://gradepro.org/.

a system for grading evidence, in order to devise a methodological approach to the development of recommendations and guidelines in healthcare.

Nine months later, in June 2004, the working group published a follow-up paper in the British Journal of Medicine. They

> present a summary of [their] approach from the perspective of a guideline user. Judgments about the strength of a recommendation require consideration of the balance between benefits and harms, the quality of the evidence, translation of the evidence into specific circumstances, and the certainty of the baseline risk. It is also important to consider costs (resource utilisation) before making a recommendation. Inconsistencies among systems for grading the quality of evidence and the strength of recommendations reduce their potential to facilitate critical appraisal and improve communication of these judgments [306]

Their idea was to develop a standardized system for judging the evidence from published research in order to make recommendations mainly with the goal to develop intervention guidelines. They define quality of evidence as

Definition the extent to which one can be confident that an estimate of effect is correct [306]

Right away, we see that this definition concerns *causal* relationships. Confidence in the correctness of an effect estimate requires a judgement call about the *relationship* between the variables that represent intervention and outcome, which we usually conceptualize as a causal relationship.

Regarding the outcome of their endeavor, mainly guidelines and recommendations for health care and public health, the GRADE group defines the strength of a recommendation as

Definition the extent to which one can be confident that adherence to the recommendation will do more good than harm [306]

This statement also concerns causal interactions, because it asks for a causal inference. In order to gain such confidence we need to make a prediction based on prior evidence whether the recommendation will generate (cause) more good than harm.

Apparently, both the definition of quality of evidence and the definition of the strength of evidence-based recommendations (defined as a positive risk-benefit ratio) involve judgements about causal inference and/or explanation.

The authors propose to proceed in sequential steps when making judgements about (1) the quality of evidence across studies; (2) which outcomes to include; (3) the overall quality of evidence across outcomes; (4) benefit-harm balance; and (5) the strength of the recommendations. Further, they propose to judge the quality of the available evidence in four main areas, i.e., study design (randomized versus observational) and quality, consistency across studies, and directness ("the extent to which the people, interventions, and outcome measures are similar to those of interest" [306]). The authors of the article continue along these lines, meandering between the understandable desire to capture evidence quality in a numeric system, and the obvious necessity to base the assessment of the quality of evidence on judgement calls. At the very least, these are judgement calls regarding, e.g., strong evidence for association if the relative risk estimate for that association is >2 (or <0.5), and very strong if it is >5 (or <0.2).

The authors envision a simple point system. They do not to propose a *quality of evidence scale*, but four recommendation categories: do it/don't do it, and probably do it and probably don't do it. Overall, the system seems to be well thought out, and it provides a good structure to thinking about the available evidence in the health literature on interventions. The GRADE evaluation system has since been implemented in a software, GradePro and an online version is available as well (GradePro GDT). In essence, the software helps the user to produce Cochrane reviews, i.e., systematic reviews of published evidence, mainly of intervention studies, but also of observational research.

The most comprehensive guide to the approach is probably the GRADE handbook.[3] Furthermore, the group has published a series of papers in the Journal of Clinical Epidemiology that introduces GRADE in detail [307–324] and has recently complemented that introductory series with multiple papers that focus on health equity in guideline development [325–328].

The GRADE concept and software is widely used in healthcare and public health. The World Health Organization has used it for guideline development, for example to develop the 2010 guidelines regarding antiretroviral drugs for treating pregnant women and preventing HIV infection in infants.[4]

Evidence-based decision-making systems that rely on summaries of intervention reports published in the scientific health literature seem to be evidence evaluation systems only at first glance. On closer inspection, they are basically guidelines for the review of the health literature by experts, who form decisions about the quality and value of that literature based on traditional epidemiological and biostatistical criteria, such as clearly articulated goals, interventions and outcomes, on sample size, minimization of bias, and so forth. Indeed, such systems do *not* evaluate the available information for decision-making, guideline development, and the design of recommendations. They provide help, instructions and guidelines to experts, whose decisions about what to decide and recommend may or may not be better when using such systems versus not using them. To our knowledge, no such comparison or validation has been performed as of the time of this writing. Meanwhile, other systems designed to evaluate the quality of systematic reviews have been developed and validated, e.g., the ROBIS (risk of bias in systematic reviews) tool appears to exhibit "fair reliability and good construct validity" [329].

The impact of evidence-grading systems such as GRADE will become apparent in due time. Meanwhile, let's revisit the issue that quality of evidence and strength

[3] available at http://gdt.guidelinedevelopment.org/app/handbook/handbook.html.

[4] http://www.who.int/hiv/pub/mtct/antiretroviral2010/en/.

of recommendation are both defined (in the context of GRADE) in terms of the validity of causal inference and explanation.

7.5 Complexity and Simplicity

Now that we have dealt with systems biology, systems medicine, and systems epidemiology in the previous section, let us briefly think through some of the issues related to system complexity versus simplicity.

7.5.1 Complexity

Complex systems are complex because their *causal* structure and function are complex. Causal function is a process. Thus, health, as a complex system, is a complex process.

Systems theory was developed in the first half of the 20th century. A system can be defined as

Definition a complex of interacting components together with the relationships among them that permit the identification of a boundary-maintaining entity or process [330].

In this definition, a *system* is a *complex* of components, the meaning of *complex* being a set of related components. The term goes back to Ludwig von Bertalanffy (1901–1972), who coined the term *general system theory*. Von Bertalanffy considered the analysis of biological systems one of the main goals of general system theory. When applied to living systems, concepts such as organization, hierarchy, and interaction phenomena provide the basis the notions of feedback loops and mechanistic processes.

The methods of classical science rely on 'reduction to components,' an approach that emphasizes the study of how one molecule, one cell, or one organ responds to a stimulus. The systems approach, on the other hand, promotes 'expansion to dynamics,' which can identify how complex sets of components behave when exposed to a complex set of influences. This emphasis on relationships between system components (rather than the components themselves) gives rise to the concept of emergence, the generation of novel phenomena at the systems level, not at the level of its isolated components in isolation. Thus, part of the "systems view" in science is that zooming out to study networks of interacting parts can better contribute to an improved understanding of the system's function and its emergent properties than zooming in on each of its components (or a few of them) in isolation.

Complexity arises in the borderland between determinism and probabilism, our two views of how the world works. In this book, we argue that the two are not mutually exclusive, but complement one another in interesting ways, describing our central theme, causal explanation.

Some parts of the world (mostly in contexts that involve inanimate objects) function in deterministic ways, while others (frequently in contexts that involve living subjects) behave in non-deterministic, probabilistic ways. This, in turn, renders perfect prediction impossible because probabilism contaminates determinism. Therefore the causal explanation of brain cancer etiology relies on the study of sets of risk factors, why the outcome of a certain brain cancer treatment is likely (but never certain) to be good, and why the odds of long term neurological sequelae of such treatment cannot be predicted with comforting certainty.

Similarly, risk estimation in the health sciences is a probabilistic concept (see Chap. 6). Two distinct ways of talking about *risk* are connected via the question, "Who is at risk?" If the answer is, "I am at risk", the risk is meant to be a dangerous place for me to be with regard to an adverse event potentially happening to me in the future (individual risk). If the answer is, "We are at risk", the risk can be quantified, as a percentage or incidence likelihood of the adverse event to happen (population risk). Both should be kept separate and the rather common communication by health care providers of percentages to individuals should be considered meaningless.

Health information systems are tools to transform health data into information that can be put to use as evidence or knowledge (or both) in the health sciences. Information can be used as evidence when it is needed in support of a claim, notion, position, intervention, or policy in health care and public health. It can also be put to use as material for tools such as decision-making processes and knowledge generation, or as feedback information for improvement of the health information systems that produced it in the first place.

The main issues related to complex systems that are relevant for our discussion are "thinking about dynamic processes, making them explicit through the formulation of dynamic conceptual models, and exploring these processes through formal models and computer simulations" [331]. The strongest motivation to tackle these issues is probably the strong belief that

> creating a healthy, sustainable future requires a fundamental shift in the way we generate, learn from, and act on evidence about the delayed and distal effects of our technologies, policies, and institutions. The reductionist program of ever-finer specialization is no longer sufficient [332]

Interestingly, despite the fact that integration is very much en vogue, some have argued that the different functions and organizational features of medicine for individuals and public health activities for populations justifies the notion that

> the overall system can be dramatically improved by establishing 2 separate but linked systems with distinct organizational forms: (a) a high-efficiency system performing large-scale repetitive tasks such as screening tests, inoculations, and generic health care, and (b) a high-complexity system treating complex medical problems of individual patients. [333]

We strongly disagree with this notion, because it suggests that population health and primary care tasks are not complex, hence mainly in need of effectiveness-makers, while solving complex health problems in individuals needs complex problem-solving methods. Instead, we argue that both areas of healthcare; i.e., both clinical/medical and population/prevention issues are in need of both efficiency improvement and complex problem solving. Moreover, although we agree that short term goals in both areas of healthcare are different, their long term goal of improving the human condition requires their integration at the information science back end. Sound and efficient causal reasoning is, in our opinion, a very important part of that process.

7.5.2 *Simplicity*

Complex systems thinking is considered in epidemiology as in other sciences [334]. It has long been acknowledged that illness causation is multivariable in that it is not one, but a whole host of causes that contribute to illness occurrence. Even in the area of infectious disease, once thought to be a clear-cut case of the one cause – one disease paradigm (Henle-Koch), it has become evident that sometimes getting infected doesn't suffice to get sick. For example, not all who are infected with HIV develop AIDS, even without anti-retroviral therapy. Thus, the notion of *complex disease* has become more prevalent in the medical literature: the absolute number of articles with the terms *complex disease* or *complex diseases* in the title has increased from 9 in 1990 to 72 in 2015, an eight-fold increase. During the same time, the total number of published papers has increased from 497,489 to 1,313,162, a 2.6-fold increase.

When life becomes too complex and difficult to handle, we invent tools to make it a bit easier. The wheel was invented to make transportation easier. The dishwasher was invented to make dishwashing less cumbersome, and the space-rocket was invented to make it easier to get to the moon. In the case of complex diseases, researchers have developed comprehensive data collection and analysis tools that employ highly complex algorithms such as, for example, network analysis [335]. The most prominent difficulty with such elaborate analytical strategies is that they represent a black box to the health care practitioner, and sometimes also to health researchers that are unfamiliar with them.

In its simplest form, the epidemiological method reveals a statistical *association* between exposure and outcome (see Sect. 6.3). According to the well-known caveat, "correlation does not mean causation", this association between an exposure and an outcome is *not yet* considered causal. Usually, epidemiologists want this *univariable* calculation of association to consider confounders by performing *multivariable* calculations, coherence with similar pertinent research results, good prediction of future events related to similar exposure-outcome constellations, and ultimately successful intervention.

Epidemiology makes causal inference easier by making it *simpler* to arrive at a causal conclusion about a particular exposure-outcome relationship. Epidemiologists use this simplification process in order to strip the situation of all its multivariable, multilevel complexity and they do that by relying on one assumption, the strength of the association between exposure and outcome.

We believe that the epidemiological method was developed to make causal inference in the health sciences simpler. The idea is to sidestep the complexity of illness causation down to the relationship between one risk factor and one disease. When this turns out to be a strong, statistically significant relationship, and remains such when confounders are controlled for, testing for coherence and intervention further increases confidence in the causal nature the association. This simple, straight forward approach is the epidemiological approach to causation, and has been very successful.

With reference to the Duhem-Quine *no miracles argument* [336], we propose that it is precisely the capability of the epidemiological method to simplify our thinking about illness causation that has made medicine, and arguably public health in particular, so successful in the recent century: Medical treatment and population intervention works *because of* deliberate simplification.

7.6 Summary

We started this chapter by dissecting the concept of evidence in the context of public health. In particular, we discuss three perspectives: the *target, method,* and *manipulation* perspectives. With *target* we mean the difference between individual and population perspectives, as discussed in Chap. 6. The *method* perspective simply refers to where we are coming from: epidemiology or basic laboratory science. We discuss recent developments in this area, in particular systems approaches in biology, medicine, and epidemiology and propose *systems health* as an overarching term. *Manipulation* is the perspective that distinguishes between non-interventional and interventional (experimental) research. In medicine and public health, this perspective refers to evidence that comes mainly from randomized studies, and we discuss the GRADE software system as an example of how informatics approaches are used for evidence assessment in the health sciences.

We conclude the chapter with a brief section that compares complexity and simplicity in population health science. We end with the somewhat provocative suggestion that epidemiological ways of risk estimation/causal explanation provide just enough complexity to appreciate the multivariable nature of biomedical causation scenarios, while maintaining a degree of simplicity that acknowledges the difficulties most of us have with juggling more than three variables in our heads at any given point in time. Perhaps this balance between seeing the complex and doing the simple is what has helped make modern medicine and public health a success story.

Chapter 8
Conclusion and Invite

The main point of this book is that causal inference and causal explanation are crucially important to population health informatics and data science. We hope that we have gathered in the preceding chapters material that will help improve theoretical and applied work towards better population health.

Our overall plan is reflected in the sequence of chapters and their contents. In the first chapter, we introduced the goals of public health informatics and population health science, and their relationship with philosophical approaches to causation and causal inference. In Chap. 2, we laid the foundations for health data science. Chapters 3 and 4 are hard-core philosophy chapters, organized by the philosophical subdisciplines of metaphysics and epistemology, respectively. In Chap. 5, we pick up on the topic of knowledge generation by referring to the sequence from data via information and evidence to knowledge. Chapter 6 brings us back to population health science and outlines the most important approaches to causal explanation in medicine and public health, risk estimation. We suggest that risk and causation are two ways of looking at the same thing, namely, the etiological process of illness occurrence. In Chap. 7, we put everything into perspective by outlining how evidence generated in this way can be integrated with other sources of knowledge.

We deliberately refrain from taking a prescriptive approach in this book. In particular, we do not propose or even assume that there is a straightforward and clear cut methodology that ensures the correct identification of risk factors as causes of illness occurrence. In fact, we think that causation itself is not something to be discovered in nature, but a thought model to explain the regularities we observe. Because these regularities are of very different kinds, we assume that there are also very different kinds of causation models. In the medical and population health sciences, there is a long laundry list of different kinds of causation that would need to be integrated into one overarching framework. However, we believe that this might not be beneficial, because many of the practical reasons why we should be interested in causal explanation actually require very specific knowledge of very specific mechanisms that lead to illness in individuals and populations. Therefore, we think

O. Dammann, B. Smart, *Causation in Population Health Informatics and Data Science*, https://doi.org/10.1007/978-3-319-96307-5_8

it is better to subscribe to a holistic, pluralist view of causation in the health sciences.

One way to tackle this situation is to acknowledge the presence and action of multiple kinds of causation in biology and sociology, and to develop a model of explanatory coherence that allows for the integration of many different kinds of data, information, and evidence, leading to a multifaceted kind of biosocial knowledge about illness occurrence. One of us is developing this line of thought based on Hill's heuristics (as outlined in Chap. 2), and one particular approach to explanatory coherence as provided by Paul Thagard with his ECHO model [108]. Much work remains to be done at both the computational and theoretical levels in order to turn this approach into a methodology that can be used by the population health community, in support of causal discussion and reasoning.

This book is not intended to offer a final summary of approaches to causal reasoning and inference in population health informatics. To the contrary: we see it as a first step towards a broader debate about the issues we have raised. We hope to receive feedback from both the philosophy and population health science communities in the form of constructive criticism that will help improve our thinking and contribute to the mission of medicine and public health. We encourage all readers to contact us with pertinent ideas, small or large, at <olaf.dammann@tufts.edu> and/or <bsmart@uj.ac.za>, so that we can incorporate your ideas, suggestions, and critiques in the next version of this text. Thanks very much.

References

1. Magnuson JA, Fu PC. Public health informatics and information systems, Health informatics series. New York: Springer; 2014.
2. Joshi A, Thorpe L, Waldron L. Population health informatics: driving evidence-based solutions into practice. Burlington: Jones & Bartlett Learning; 2019.
3. Tulchinsky TH, Varavikova E. The new public health. 2nd ed. Amsterdam/Boston: Elsevier/Academic Press; 2009. xxiv, 672 p.
4. Institute of Medicine (U.S.) Committee on Public Health Strategies to Improve Health. For the public's health : the role of measurement in action and accountability. Washington, D.C.: National Academies Press; 2011. xv, 188 p.
5. Kharrazi H, et al. A proposed national research and development agenda for population health informatics: summary recommendations from a national expert workshop. J Am Med Inform Assoc. 2017;24(1):2–12.
6. Friede A, Blum HL, McDonald M. Public health informatics: how information-age technology can strengthen public health. Annu Rev Public Health. 1995;16:239–52.
7. Rolka H, et al. Analytical challenges for emerging public health surveillance. MMWR Suppl. 2012;61(3):35–40.
8. Bunge M. In: Dover, editor. Causality and modern science. Cambridge: Harvard University Press; 1979.
9. Lewis D. Causation. J Philos. 1973;70:556–67.
10. Mackie JL. The cement of the universe; a study of causation (The Clarendon library of logic and philosophy), vol. 329. Oxford: Clarendon Press; 1974.
11. Salmon WC. Scientific explanation and the causal structure of the world. Princeton, NJ: Princeton University Press; 1984. xiv, 305 p.
12. Eells E. Probabilistic causality. Cambridge, UK: Cambridge University Press; 1991.
13. Dowe P. Physical causation. Cambridge studies in probability, induction, and decision theory. Cambridge/New York: Cambridge University Press; 2000. ix, 224 p.
14. Cartwright N. Hunting causes and using them : approaches in philosophy and economics. Cambridge/New York: Cambridge University Press; 2007. x, 270 p.
15. Eden AH. Three paradigms of computer science. Mind Mach. 2007;17(2):135–67.
16. Tolentino H, et al. Case-based learning in public health informatics. In: Magnuson JA, Fu PC, editors. Public health informatics and information systems. London: Springer; 2014. p. 489–510.
17. Evans AS. Causation and disease – a chronological journey. New York/London: Plenum; 1993.
18. Carter KC. The rise of causal concepts of disease: case histories. Farnham: Ashgate Publishing; 2003.
19. Thagard P. How scientists explain disease. Princeton: Princeton University Press; 1999.

O. Dammann, B. Smart, *Causation in Population Health Informatics and Data Science*, https://doi.org/10.1007/978-3-319-96307-5

20. Miettinen OS, Flegel KM. Elementary concepts of medicine: V. Disease: one of the main subtypes of illness. J Eval Clin Pract. 2003;9(3):321–3.
21. Dammann O. The etiological stance: explaining illness occurrence. Perspect Biol Med. 2017;60(2):151–65.
22. Miettinen OS. Theoretical epidemiology. New York: John Wiley & Sons; 1985.
23. Rothman KJ, Greenland S. Modern epidemiology. 2nd ed. Philadelphia: Lippincott-Raven; 1998.
24. Schulte PA, Perera FP. Molecular epidemiology. Principles and practices. San Diego: Academic; 1993.
25. Khoury MJ, Beaty TH, Cohen BH. Fundamentals of genetic epidemiology. Oxford: Oxford University Press; 1993.
26. Khoury MJ, et al., editors. Human genome epidemiology. Oxford: Oxford University Press; 2010.
27. Rothman KJ. Modern epidemiology. Boston: Little, Brown & Company; 1986.
28. Savitz DA. Interpreting epidemiologic evidence. Oxford: Oxford University Press; 2003.
29. Yerushalmy J, Palmer CE. On the methodology of investigations of etiologic factors in chronic diseases. J Chronic Dis. 1959;10(1):27–40.
30. Sartwell PE. On the methodology of investigations of etiologic factors in chronic diseases – further comments. J Chronic Dis. 1960;11:61–3.
31. Lilienfeld AM. On the methodology of investigations of etiologic factors in chronic diseases: some comments. J Chronic Dis. 1959;10(1):41–6.
32. Hill AB. The environment and disease: association or causation? Proc R Soc Med. 1965;58:295–300.
33. Rothman KJ. Causes. Am J Epidemiol. 1976;104:87–92.
34. Susser M. Judgement and causal inference: criteria in epidemiologic studies. Am J Epidemiol. 1977;105(1):1–15.
35. Evans AS. Causation and disease: a chronological journey. Am J Epidemiol. 1978;108(4):249–58.
36. Weed DL. On the logic of causal inference. Am J Epidemiol. 1986;123(6):965–79.
37. Pearce N. White swans, black ravens, and lame ducks: necessary and sufficient causes in epidemiology. Epidemiology. 1990;1(1):47–50.
38. Susser M. What is a cause and how do we know one? A grammar for pragmatic epidemiology. Am J Epidemiol. 1991;133:635–48.
39. Rizzi DA, Pedersen SA. Causality in medicine: towards a theory and terminology. Theor Med. 1992;13(3):233–54.
40. Renton A. Epidemiology and causation: a realist view. J Epidemiol Community Health. 1994;48(1):79–85.
41. Krieger N. Epidemiology and the web of causation: has anyone seen the spider? Soc Sci Med. 1994;39(7):887–903.
42. Rizzi DA. Causal reasoning and the diagnostic process. Theor Med. 1994;15(3):315–33.
43. Rubin DB. Estimating causal effects from large data sets using propensity scores. Ann Intern Med. 1997;127(8 Pt 2):757–63.
44. Samuels SW. Philosophic perspectives: community, communications, and occupational disease causation. Int J Health Serv. 1998;28(1):153–64.
45. Philippe P, Mansi O. Nonlinearity in the epidemiology of complex health and disease processes. Theor Med Bioeth. 1998;19(6):591–607.
46. Greenland S, Pearl J, Robins JM. Causal diagrams for epidemiologic research. Epidemiology. 1999;10(1):37–48.
47. Flier FJ, de Vries Robbé PF. Nosology and causal necessity; the relation between defining a disease and discovering its necessary cause. Theor Med Bioeth. 1999;20(6):577–88.
48. Scheutz F, Poulsen S. Determining causation in epidemiology. Community Dent Oral Epidemiol. 1999;27(3):161–70.
49. Little RJ, Rubin DB. Causal effects in clinical and epidemiological studies via potential outcomes: concepts and analytical approaches. Annu Rev Public Health. 2000;21:121–45.
50. Parascandola M, Weed DL. Causation in epidemiology. J Epidemiol Community Health. 2001;55(12):905–12.
51. Robins JM. Data, design, and background knowledge in etiologic inference. Epidemiology. 2001;12(3):313–20.

52. Greenland S, Brumback B. An overview of relations among causal modelling methods. Int J Epidemiol. 2002;31(5):1030–7.
53. Maldonado G, Greenland S. Estimating causal effects. Int J Epidemiol. 2002;31(2):422–9.
54. Doll R. Proof of causality: deduction from epidemiological observation. Perspect Biol Med. 2002;45(4):499–515.
55. Dawid AP. Probability, causality and the empirical world: a Bayes-de Finetti-Popper-Borel synthesis. Stat Sci. 2004;19(1):44–57.
56. Hernán MA. A definition of causal effect for epidemiological research. J Epidemiol Community Health. 2004;58(4):265–71.
57. Raisanen U, et al. The causation of disease – the practical and ethical consequences of competing explanations. Med Health Care Philos. 2006;9(3):293–306.
58. Dekkers W, Rikkert MO. What is a genetic cause? The example of Alzheimer's disease. Med Health Care Philos. 2006;9(3):273–84.
59. Petersen ML, Sinisi SE, van der Laan MJ. Estimation of direct causal effects. Epidemiology. 2006;17(3):276–84.
60. Hernan MA, Robins JM. Estimating causal effects from epidemiologic data. J Epidemiol Community Health. 2006;60:578–86.
61. Weed DL. Truth, epidemiology, and general causation. Brooklyn Law Rev. 2008;73(3):943–57.
62. Cartwright N. Causation: one word, many things. Philos Sci. 2004;71:805–19.
63. Illari PM, Russo F. Causality: philosophical theory meets scientific practice. 1st ed. Oxford: Oxford University Press; 2014. xiv, 310 p.
64. Susser MW. Causal thinking in the health sciences – concepts and strategies of epidemiology. New York/London/Toronto: Oxford University Press; 1973.
65. Weed DL. On the use of causal criteria. Int J Epidemiol. 1997;26(6):1137–41.
66. Greenland S. Probability logic and probabilistic induction. Epidemiology. 1998;9(3):322–32.
67. Greenland S. Relation of probability of causation to relative risk and doubling dose: a methodologic error that has become a social problem. Am J Public Health. 1999;89(8):1166–9.
68. Salmon WC. Probabilistic causality. In: Sosa E, Tooley M, editors. Causation. Oxford: Oxford University Press; 1993. p. 137–53.
69. Salmon WC. Causality and explanation. New York: Oxford University Press; 1998. xiv, 434 p.
70. Woodward J. Making things happen – a theory of causal explanation. Oxford/New York: Oxford University Press; 2003.
71. Woodward J. Agency and interventionist theories. In: Beebee H, Hitchcock C, Menzies P, editors. The Oxford handbook of causation. Oxford: OUP; 2009. p. 234–62.
72. Casini L, et al. Models for prediction, explanation and control: recursive Bayesian networks. Theoria. 2011;11(1):5–33.
73. Clarke B, et al. Mechanisms and the evidence hierarchy. Topoi. 2014;33(2):339–60.
74. Clarke B, et al. The evidence that evidence-based medicine omits. Prev Med. 2013;57(6):745–7.
75. Illari P, Williamson J. What is a mechanism? Thinking about mechanisms across the sciences. Eur J Phil Sci. 2012;2:119–35.
76. Nagl S, Williams M, Williamson J. Objective Bayesian nets for systems modelling and prognosis in breast cancer. In: Holmes D, Jain LC, editors. Innovations in Bayesian networks: theory and applications, vol. 156: Springer; 2008. p. 131–67.
77. Russo F, Williamson J. Interpreting causality in the health sciences. Int Stud Philos Sci. 2007;21(2):157–70.
78. Russo F, Williamson J. Generic versus single-case causality: the case of autopsy. Eur J Philos Sci. 2011;1:47–69.
79. Broadbent A. Inferring causation in epidemiology: mechanisms, black boxes, and contrasts. In: Illari PM, Russo F, Williamson J, editors. Causality in the sciences. Oxford: Oxford University Press; 2011. p. 45–69.
80. Broadbent A. Philosophy of epidemiology. New directions in the philosophy of science. Houndmills, UK: Palgrave Macmillan; 2013.
81. Vandenbroucke JP, Broadbent A, Pearce N. Causality and causal inference in epidemiology: the need for a pluralistic approach. Int J Epidemiol. 2016;45(6):1776–86.
82. Loudon I. Ignaz Phillip Semmelweis' studies of death in childbirth. J R Soc Med. 2013;106(11):461–3.

83. Paneth N. Assessing the contributions of John snow to epidemiology: 150 years after removal of the broad street pump handle. Epidemiology. 2004;15(5):514–6.
84. Berthelsen PG. John Snow – three original insights, one misconception, and an overdue obituary. Acta Anaesthesiol Scand. 2017;61(5):566–71.
85. Steurer J, Bachmann LM, Miettinen OS. Etiology in a taxonomy of illnesses. Eur J Epidemiol. 2006;21(2):85–9.
86. Evans AS. Causation and disease: the Henle-Koch postulates revisited. Yale J Biol Med. 1976;49(2):175–95.
87. Fujimura JH, Chou DY. Dissent in science: styles of scientific practice and the controversy over the cause of AIDS. Soc Sci Med. 1994;38(8):1017–36.
88. Choudhary SK, et al. Low immune activation despite high levels of pathogenic human immunodeficiency virus type 1 results in long-term asymptomatic disease. J Virol. 2007;81(16):8838–42.
89. Buck C. Popper's philosophy for epidemiologists. Int J Epidemiol. 1975;4(3):159–68.
90. Pearce N, Crawford-Brown D. Critical discussion in epidemiology: problems with the Popperian approach. J Clin Epidemiol. 1989;42(3):177–84.
91. Leviton A. Single-cause attribution. Dev Med Child Neurol. 1987;29(6):805–7.
92. Blair E, Stanley F. When can cerebral palsy be prevented? The generation of causal hypotheses by multivariate analysis of a case-control study. Paediatr Perinat Epidemiol. 1993;7(3):272–301.
93. Halloran ME, Struchiner CJ. Causal inference in infectious diseases. Epidemiology. 1995;6(2):142–51.
94. Dowe P, Noordhof P, editors. Cause and chance. London/New York: Routledge; 2004.
95. Rothman KJ, et al. Causation and causal inference. In: Rothman KJ, Greenland S, Lash TL, editors. Modern epidemiology. Philadelphia: Lippincott Williams & Wilkins; 2008. p. 5–31.
96. Skrabanek P. The emptiness of the black box. Epidemiology. 1994;5(5):553–5.
97. Rorty R. A world without substances or essences. In: Philosophy and social hope. London: Penguin; 1999. p. 47–71.
98. Mumford S, Anjum RL. Getting causes from powers. Oxford/New York: Oxford University Press; 2011. xvi, 254 p.
99. Morabia A. On the origin of Hill's causal criteria. Epidemiology. 1991;2(5):367–9.
100. Dammann O, Leviton A. Perinatal brain damage causation. Dev Neurosci. 2007;29(4–5):280–8.
101. Maclure M. Multivariate refutation of aetiological hypotheses in non-experimental epidemiology. Int J Epidemiol. 1990;19(4):782–7.
102. Dammann O, Karmaus W. Fletcher's paradox. Epidemiology. 1992;3(6):540–2.
103. Beebee H, Hitchcock C, Menzies PC. The Oxford handbook of causation. Oxford: Oxford University Press; 2009. xv, 790 p.
104. Illari PM, Russo F, Williamson J. Causality in the sciences. Oxford/New York: Oxford University Press; 2011. xiii, 938 p.
105. Dworkin MS, et al. An outbreak of varicella among children attending preschool and elementary school in Illinois. Clin Infect Dis. 2002;35(1):102–4.
106. Morabia A. Hume, mill, hill, and the sui generis epidemiologic approach to causal inference. Am J Epidemiol. 2013;178(10):1526–32.
107. Ioannidis JP. Exposure-wide epidemiology: revisiting Bradford Hill. Stat Med. 2016;35:1749–62.
108. Dammann O. Hill's heuristics and explanatory coherentism in epidemiology. Am J Epidemiol. 2018;187(1):1–6.
109. Cao LB. Data science: challenges and directions. Commun ACM. 2017;60(8):59–68.
110. Ohno-Machado L. Data science and informatics: when it comes to biomedical data, is there a real distinction? J Am Med Inform Assoc. 2013;20(6):1009.
111. Floridi L. Artificial intelligence's new frontier: artificial companions and the fourth revolution. Metaphilosophy. 2008;39(4–5):651–5.
112. Floridi L. The philosophy of information. Oxford/New York: Oxford University Press; 2011. xviii, 405 p.

113. Tedre M. Computing as a science: a survey of competing viewpoints. Mind Mach. 2011;21(3):361–87.
114. Haux R. Medical informatics: past, present, future. Int J Med Inform. 2010;79(9):599–610.
115. Dixon BE, Kharrazi H, Lehmann HP. Public health and epidemiology informatics: recent research and trends in the United States. Yearb Med Inform. 2015;10(1):199–206.
116. Heller RF. Evidence for population health. Oxford/New York: Oxford University Press; 2005. xii, 126 p.
117. Shortliffe EH, Cimino JJ. Biomedical informatics : computer applications in health care and biomedicine, Health informatics series. 3rd ed. New York: Springer; 2006. xxvi, 1037 p.
118. Porta MS, International Epidemiological Association. A dictionary of epidemiology. 5th ed. Oxford/New York: Oxford University Press; 2008. xxiv, 289 p.
119. Savel TG, et al. The role of public health informatics in enhancing public health surveillance. MMWR Surveill Summ. 2012;61(Suppl):20–4.
120. Buehler JW, Centers for Disease, and Prevention. CDC's vision for public health surveillance in the 21st century. Introduction. MMWR Surveill Summ. 2012;61(Suppl):1–2.
121. Teutsch SM. Considerations in planning a surveillance system. In: Lee LM, et al., editors. Principles & practice of public health surveillance. Oxford: Oxford University Press; 2010. p. 18–31.
122. Thacker SB, et al. Public health surveillance in the United States: evolution and challenges. MMWR Surveill Summ. 2012;61(Suppl):3–9.
123. Lee LM. In: Lee LM, et al., editors. Principles & practice of public health surveillance. 3rd ed. Oxford/New York: Oxford University Press; 2010. xiv, 443 p.
124. Sullivan PS, et al. Analyzing and interpreting public health surveillance data. In: Lee LM, et al., editors. Principles & practice of public health surveillance. Oxford: Oxford University Press; 2010. p. 88–145.
125. Kirch W. Encyclopedia of public health. New York: Springer; 2008.
126. Savitz DA, Poole C, Miller WC. Reassessing the role of epidemiology in public health. Am J Public Health. 1999;89(8):1158–61.
127. MacMahon B, Pugh TF. Epidemiology; principles and methods. 1st ed. Boston: Little, 1970. ix, 376 p.
128. Thrusfield MV. Veterinary epidemiology. London/Boston: Butterworths; 1986. viii, 280 p.
129. Kuznetsov V, et al. How bioinformatics influences health informatics: usage of biomolecular sequences, expression profiles and automated microscopic image analyses for clinical needs and public health. Health Inf Sci Syst. 2013;1:2.
130. Glass TA, et al. Causal inference in public health. Annu Rev Public Health. 2013;34:61–75.
131. Cochrane AL. Effectiveness and efficiency: random reflections on health services. In: The rock carling fellowship. London: Nuffield Provincial Hospitals Trust; 1972. xi, 92 p.
132. Evidence-Based Medicine Working Group. Evidence-based medicine. A new approach to teaching the practice of medicine. JAMA. 1992;268(17):2420–5.
133. Sackett DL, et al. Evidence based medicine: what it is and what it isn't. BMJ. 1996;312(7023):71–2.
134. Timmermans S, Mauck A. The promises and pitfalls of evidence-based medicine. Health Aff (Millwood). 2005;24(1):18–28.
135. Milstein RL, Wetterhall SF. Framework for program evaluation in public health. MMWR Recomm Rep. 1999;48(RR-11):1–40.
136. Bataille V, et al. Exposure to the sun and sunbeds and the risk of cutaneous melanoma in the UK: a case-control study. Eur J Cancer. 2004;40(3):429–35.
137. Bodei C, Bracciali A, Chiarugi D. On deducing causality in metabolic networks. BMC Bioinformatics. 2008;9:S8.
138. Cartwright N. Nature's capacities and their measurement. Oxford/New York: Clarendon Press/Oxford University Press; 1989. x, 268 p.
139. Vamathevan J, Birney E. A review of recent advances in translational bioinformatics: bridges from biology to medicine. Yearb Med Inform. 2017;26(1):178–87.
140. Van Neste L, Van Criekinge W. We are all individuals. Bioinformatics in the personalized medicine era. Cell Oncol. 2015;38(1):29–37.

141. Chen ML, et al. Placenta microbiology and histology and the risk for severe retinopathy of prematurity. Invest Ophthalmol Vis Sci. 2011;52:7052–8.
142. Dammann O, et al. Systems epidemiology: what's in a name? Online J Public Health Inform. 2014;6(3):e198.
143. Rorty R. The linguistic turn; recent essays in philosophical method, vol. 393. Chicago: University of Chicago Press; 1967.
144. Mill JS. A system of logic. 4th ed. London: John W. Parker & Son; 1856.
145. Stampfer MJ, et al. Postmenopausal estrogen therapy and cardiovascular disease. Ten-year follow-up from the nurses' health study. N Engl J Med. 1991;325(11):756–62.
146. Hulley S, et al. Randomized trial of estrogen plus progestin for secondary prevention of coronary heart disease in postmenopausal women. Heart and Estrogen/progestin Replacement Study (HERS) Research Group. JAMA. 1998;280(7):605–13.
147. Rossouw JE, et al. Risks and benefits of estrogen plus progestin in healthy postmenopausal women – principal results from the women's health initiative randomized controlled trial. JAMA-J Am Med Assoc. 2002;288(3):321–33.
148. Lawlor DA, Smith GD, Ebrahim S. Socioeconomic position and hormone replacement therapy use: explaining the discrepancy in evidence from observational and randomized controlled trials. Am J Public Health. 2004;94(12):2149–54.
149. Vandenbroucke JP. The HRT controversy: observational studies and RCTs fall in line. Lancet. 2009;373(9671):1233–5.
150. Khoury MJ. Genetic epidemiology. In: Rothman KJ, Greenland S, editors. Modern epidemiology. Philadelphia: Lippincott-Raven; 1998. p. 609–21.
151. Hume DA. In: Beauchamp TL, editor. An enquiry concerning human understanding. Oxford: Oxford University Press; 1999.
152. Hitchcock C. Of Humean bondage. Br J Philos Sci. 2003;54:1–25.
153. Kapetanovic IM, Rosenfeld S, Izmirlian G. Overview of commonly used bioinformatics methods and their applications. Ann N Y Acad Sci. 2004;1020:10–21.
154. Wolkenhauer O, Green S. The search for organizing principles as a cure against reductionism in systems medicine. FEBS J. 2013;280(23):5938–48.
155. Rothman KJ. Epidemiology: an introduction. Oxford: Oxford University Press; 2012.
156. Smart B. Concepts and causes in the philosophy of disease. Basingstoke/New York: Palgrave pivot/Palgrave Macmillan; 2016. ix, 100 p.
157. Fuller J. What are chronic diseases? Synthese. 2018;195:3197–220.
158. Low M. A novel clinical framework: the use of dispositions in clinical practice. A person centred approach. J Eval Clin Pract. 2017;23(5):1062–70.
159. Smart B. On the classification of diseases. Theor Med Bioeth. 2014;35(4):251–69.
160. Schroeder SA. Rethinking health: healthy or healthier than? Br J Philos Sci. 2013;64(1):131–59.
161. Whitbeck C. Causation in medicine – disease entity model. Philos Sci. 1977;44(4):619–37.
162. Bensing J. Bridging the gap. The separate worlds of evidence-based medicine and patient-centered medicine. Patient Educ Couns. 2000;39(1):17–25.
163. Ichikawa JJ, Steup M. The analysis of knowledge. The stanford Encyclopedia of philosophy 2013 03/07/2014. Available from: http://plato.stanford.edu/archives/fall2013/entries/knowledge-analysis/.
164. Stegenga J. Medical nihilism. New York: Oxford University Press; 2018. pages cm.
165. Martí-Ibáñez F. A prelude to medical history. New York: MD Publications; 1961. p. 253.
166. Hippocrates, et al. Hippocratic writings (pelican classics). New ed. Harmondsworth/New York: Penguin; 1978. 380 p.
167. Cartwright N. Will this policy work for you? Predicting effectiveness better: how philosophy helps. Philos Sci. 2012;79(5):973–89.
168. Ioannidis JP. Why most published research findings are false. PLoS Med. 2005;2(8):e124.
169. Van Fraassen BC. Laws and symmetry. Oxford/New York: Oxford University Press; 1989. xv, 395 p.

170. Weed DW. In: Rothman KJ, editor. Causal criteria and Popperian refutation, in Causal inference. Chestnut Hill: Epidemiology Resources Inc.; 1988. p. 15–32.
171. Phillips CV, Goodman KJ. Causal criteria and counterfactuals; nothing more (or less) than scientific common sense. Emerg Themes Epidemiol. 2006;3:5.
172. Poole C. Causal values. Epidemiology. 2001;12(2):139–41.
173. Rothman KJ, Greenland S. Hill's criteria for causality. In: Encyclopedia of biostatistics, online; 2005.
174. Blackburn H, Labarthe D. Stories from the evolution of guidelines for causal inference in epidemiologic associations: 1953-1965. Am J Epidemiol. 2012;176(12):1071–7.
175. Lucas RM, McMichael AJ. Association or causation: evaluating links between environment and disease. Bull World Health Organ. 2005;83(10):792–5.
176. Kim Y-H, et al. Delayed choice quantum eraser. Phys Rev Lett. 2000;84(1):1.
177. Shadish WR, Cook TD, Campbell DT. Experimental and quasi-experimental designs for generalized causal inference. Boston: Houghton Mifflin; 2001. xxi, 623 p.
178. Worrall J. Why there's no cause to randomize. Br J Philos Sci. 2007;58(3):451–88.
179. Burch PR. The surgeon general's epidemiologic criteria for causality. A critique. J Chronic Dis. 1983;36(12):821–36.
180. United States. Surgeon General's Advisory Committee on Smoking and Health., Smoking and health; report of the advisory committee to the Surgeon General of the Public Health Service. Public Health Service publication no 1103. 1964, Washington: U.S. Dept. of Health, Education, and Welfare, Public Health Service; for sale by the Superintendent of Documents, U.S. Govt. Print. Off. xvii, 387 p.
181. Gettier J. Is justified true belief knowledge? Analysis. 1963;23(6):121–3.
182. Goldman AI. A causal theory of knowing. J Philos. 1967;64(12):357–72.
183. Conee EB, Feldman R. Evidentialism : essays in epistemology, vol. 321. Oxford/New York: Oxford University Press; 2004.
184. Hintikka J. Knowing that one knows reviewed. Synthese. 1970;21(2):141–62.
185. Armstrong DM. Belief, truth and knowledge. London: Cambridge University Press; 1973. ix, 228 p.
186. Solomon M. Making medical knowledge. 1st ed. Oxford: Oxford University Press; 2015. xiii, 261 p.
187. Yasnoff WA, O'Carroll PW, Friede A. Public health informatics and the health information infrastructure. In: Shortliffe EH, Cimino JJ, editors. Biomedical informatics. New York: Springer; 2006. p. 537–63.
188. Revere D, et al. Understanding the information needs of public health practitioners: a literature review to inform design of an interactive digital knowledge management system. J Biomed Inform. 2007;40(4):410–21.
189. Ackoff RL. From data to wisdom. J Appl Syst Anal. 1989;16.3–9.
190. Rowley J. The wisdom hierarchy: representations of the DIKW hierarchy. J Inf Sci. 2007;33(2):163–80.
191. Chaffey D, Wood SJ. Business information management: improving perfomance using information systems. Upper Saddle River: Prentice Hall; 2005.
192. Choo CW. The knowing organization: how organizations use information to construct meaning, create knowledge and make decisions. Int J Inf Manag. 1996;16(5):329–40.
193. Heller RF, Page J. A population perspective to evidence based medicine: evidence for population health. J Epidemiol Community Health. 2002;56(1):45–7.
194. Holland PW. Statistics and causal inference. J Am Stat Assoc. 1986;81(396):945–60.
195. Mensah E, Goderre JL. Data sources and data tools. In: Magnuson JA, Fu PC, editors. Public health informatics and information systems. London: Springer; 2014. p. 107–31.
196. Audi R. The Cambridge dictionary of philosophy. 2nd ed. Cambridge/New York: Cambridge University Press; 1999. xxxv, 1001 p.
197. Brownson RC, Fielding JE, Maylahn CM. Evidence-based public health: a fundamental concept for public health practice. Annu Rev Public Health. 2009;30:175–201.

198. Viehbeck SM, Petticrew M, Cummins S. Old myths, new myths: challenging myths in public health. Am J Public Health. 2015;105(4):665–9.
199. Beer KD, et al. Surveillance for waterborne disease outbreaks associated with drinking water – United States, 2011-2012. MMWR Morb Mortal Wkly Rep. 2015;64(31):842–8.
200. Lucey KG. On knowing and the known : introductory readings in epistemology. Amherst: Prometheus Books; 1996. 437 p.
201. Johns ML. Information management for health professions, The health information management series. 2nd ed. Albany: Delmar Thomson Learning; 2002. xx, 390 p.
202. Fleck L. Genesis and development of a scientific fact. Chicago: University of Chicago Press; 1979. xxviii, 203 p.
203. Bellinger DC. Lead contamination in flint – an abject failure to protect public health. N Engl J Med. 2016;374(12):1101–3.
204. Dean K. Creating a new knowledge base for the new public health. J Epidemiol Community Health. 1994;48(3):217–9.
205. Eriksson C. Learning and knowledge-production for public health: a review of approaches to evidence-based public health. Scand J Public Health. 2000;28(4):298–308.
206. Russell SJ, Norvig P. Artificial intelligence: a modern approach. Upper Saddle River: Prentice Hall; 2010.
207. Best A, et al. Knowledge integration: conceptualizing communications in cancer control systems. Patient Educ Couns. 2008;71(3):319–27.
208. Greenhalgh T, Wieringa S. Is it time to drop the knowledge translation metaphor? A critical literature review. J R Soc Med. 2011;104(12):501–9.
209. Green LW, et al. Diffusion theory and knowledge dissemination, utilization, and integration in public health. Annu Rev Public Health. 2009;30:151–74.
210. Khoury MJ, et al. Knowledge integration at the center of genomic medicine. Genet Med. 2012;14(7):643–7.
211. Murray KS, Porter BW. Developing a tool for knowledge integration – initial results. Int J Man Mach Stud. 1990;33(4):373–83.
212. Kamper-Jorgensen F. Knowledge-base, evidence and evaluation in public health. Scand J Public Health. 2000;28(4):241–3.
213. Cartwright N. Are RCTs the gold standard? BioSocieties. 2007;2(1):11–20.
214. Sujansky W. Heterogeneous database integration in biomedicine. J Biomed Inform. 2001;34(4):285–98.
215. Louie B, et al. Data integration and genomic medicine. J Biomed Inform. 2007;40(1):5–16.
216. Galperin MY, Rigden DJ, Fernandez-Suarez XM. The 2015 nucleic acids research database issue and molecular biology database collection. Nucleic Acids Res. 2015;43(Database issue):D1–5.
217. Nsoesie EO, Brownstein JS. Computational approaches to influenza surveillance: beyond timeliness. Cell Host Microbe. 2015;17(3):275–8.
218. Wolkenhauer O. Why model? Front Physiol. 2014;5:21.
219. Dammann O, Follett P. Toward multi-scale computational modeling in developmental disability research. Neuropediatrics. 2011;42(3):90–6.
220. Wolkenhauer O, et al. Enabling multiscale modeling in systems medicine. Genome Med. 2014;6(3):21.
221. Wolkenhauer O, et al. The road from systems biology to systems medicine. Pediatr Res. 2013;73(4 Pt 2):502–7.
222. Feitelson DG. From repeatability to reproducibility and corroboration. ACM SIGOPS Oper Syst Rev. 2015;49(1):3–11.
223. Malmfors T, Rosing H. Introduction – risk from a philosophy of science point of view. Toxicology. 2002;181-182:109–13.
224. Ropeik D, Gray G. Risk : a practical guide for deciding what's really safe and what's dangerous in the world around you. Boston: Houghton Mifflin; 2002. 485 p.
225. Slovic P. Perception of risk. Science. 1987;236(4799):280–5.

226. Holton GA. Defining risk. Financ Anal J. 2004;60(6):19–25.
227. Rockhill B. The privatization of risk. Am J Public Health. 2001;91(3):365–8.
228. Li G, et al. Age, flight experience, and risk of crash involvement in a cohort of professional pilots. Am J Epidemiol. 2003;157(10):874–80.
229. Rockhill B, Kawachi I, Colditz GA. Individual risk prediction and population-wide disease prevention. Epidemiol Rev. 2000;22(1):176–80.
230. Grossi E. Medical concepts related to individual risk are better explained with plausibility rather than probability. BMC Cardiovasc Disord. 2005;5:31.
231. Rothwell PM, et al. Treating individuals 3: from subgroups to individuals: general principles and the example of carotid endarterectomy. Lancet. 2005;365(9455):256–65.
232. Dammann O, et al. Bronchopulmonary dysplasia is not associated with ultrasound-defined cerebral white matter damage in preterm newborns. Pediatr Res. 2004;55:319–25.
233. Tolsma KW, et al. Neonatal bacteremia and retinopathy of prematurity: the ELGAN study. Arch Ophthalmol. 2011;129(12):1555–63.
234. Pearson K. The grammar of science. 2nd ed. London: A. and C. Black; 1900. xviii, 548 p.
235. Kovesdy CP, Kalantar-Zadeh K. Observational studies versus randomized controlled trials: avenues to causal inference in nephrology. Adv Chronic Kidney Dis. 2012;19(1):11–8.
236. Flanagan R, Dammann O. The epistemological weight of randomized-controlled trials depend on their results. Perspect Biol Med. (in press).
237. Education, T.I.U.f.H.P. The evidence of health promotion effectiveness. Shaping public health in a New Europe. Brussels: European Commission DGV; 1999.
238. Braveman P. Combining forces against inequity and poverty rather than splitting hairs. Bull World Health Organ. 2000;78(1):78–9.
239. Auffray C, et al. From functional genomics to systems biology: concepts and practices. C R Biol. 2003;326(10–11):879–92.
240. Hood L. Systems biology: integrating technology, biology, and computation. Mech Ageing Dev. 2003;124(1):9–16.
241. Kitano H. Computational systems biology. Nature. 2002;420(6912):206–10.
242. Wolkenhauer O. Systems biology: the reincarnation of systems theory applied in biology? Brief Bioinform. 2001;2(3):258–70.
243. Apweiler R, et al. Whither systems medicine? Exp Mol Med. 2018;50(3):e453.
244. Auffray C, Chen Z, Hood L. Systems medicine: the future of medical genomics and healthcare. Genome Med. 2009;1(1):2.
245. Hood L, Flores M. A personal view on systems medicine and the emergence of proactive P4 medicine: predictive, preventive, personalized and participatory. N Biotechnol. 2012;29(6):613–24.
246. Comas I, Gagneux S. A role for systems epidemiology in tuberculosis research. Trends Microbiol. 2011;19(10):492–500.
247. Cornelis MC, Hu FB. Systems epidemiology: a new direction in nutrition and metabolic disease research. Curr Nutr Rep. 2013;2(4):225–35.
248. Joffe M, et al. Causal diagrams in systems epidemiology. Emerg Themes Epidemiol. 2012;9(1):1.
249. Lund E, Dumeaux V. Systems epidemiology in cancer. Cancer Epidemiol Biomark Prev. 2008;17(11):2954–7.
250. Engel GL. The need for a new medical model: a challenge for biomedicine. Science. 1977;196(4286):129–36.
251. Engel GL. The clinical application of the biopsychosocial model. Am J Psychiatry. 1980;137(5):535–44.
252. Fava GA, Sonino N. The biopsychosocial model thirty years later. Psychother Psychosom. 2008;77(1):1–2.
253. Bertalanffy LV. General system theory; foundations, development, applications. New York: George Braziller; 1968. p. xv, 289 p.
254. Machamer PK, Darden L, Craver CF. Thinking about mechanisms. Philos Sci. 2000;67:1–25.

255. Bechtel W. Mechanism and biological explanation. Philos Sci. 2011;78:533–57.
256. Epstein JM. Why model? J Artif Soc Soc Simul. 2008;11(4):12.
257. Andrade MA, Sander C. Bioinformatics: from genome data to biological knowledge. Curr Opin Biotechnol. 1997;8(6):675–83.
258. Thomas DC. The need for a systematic approach to complex pathways in molecular epidemiology. Cancer Epidemiol Biomark Prev. 2005;14(3):557–9.
259. Baxevanis AD, Ouellette BF. Bioinformatics. New York: Wiley; 2001.
260. Quackenbush J. Microarray analysis and tumor classification. N Engl J Med. 2006;354(23):2463–72.
261. Kohane IS, Butte A. Bioinformatics. In: Elston R, Olson J, Palmer L, editors. Biostatistical genetics and genetic epidemiology. Chichester: Wiley; 2002.
262. Wiley HS, Shvartsman SY, Lauffenburger DA. Computational modeling of the EGF-receptor system: a paradigm for systems biology. Trends Cell Biol. 2003;13(1):43–50.
263. Oda K, et al. A comprehensive pathway map of epidermal growth factor receptor signaling. Mol Syst Biol. 2005;1:2005 0010.
264. Oda K, Kitano H. A comprehensive map of the toll-like receptor signaling network. Mol Syst Biol. 2006;2:2006 0015.
265. Noble D. Modeling the heart. Physiology (Bethesda). 2004;19:191–7.
266. Federoff HJ, Gostin LO. Evolving from reductionism to holism: is there a future for systems medicine? JAMA. 2009;302(9):994–6.
267. Hood L, Balling R, Auffray C. Revolutionizing medicine in the 21st century through systems approaches. Biotechnol J. 2012;7(8):992–1001.
268. Rehm M, et al. Wither systems medicine? Exp Mol Med. (in press).
269. Tian Q, Price ND, Hood L. Systems cancer medicine: towards realization of predictive, preventive, personalized and participatory (P4) medicine. J Intern Med. 2012;271(2):111–21.
270. Bates S. Progress towards personalized medicine. Drug Discov Today. 2010;15(3–4):115–20.
271. Chan IS, Ginsburg GS. Personalized medicine: progress and promise. Annu Rev Genomics Hum Genet. 2011;12:217–44.
272. Nersting J, Borst L, Schmiegelow K. Challenges in implementing individualized medicine illustrated by antimetabolite therapy of childhood acute lymphoblastic leukemia. Clin Proteomics. 2011;8(1):8.
273. Collins FS, et al. A vision for the future of genomics research. Nature. 2003;422(6934):835–47.
274. Frenk J. The new public health. Annu Rev Public Health. 1993;14:469–90.
275. Schulte PA. A conceptual and historical framework for molecular epidemiology. In: Schulte PA, Perera FP, editors. Molecular epidemiology – principles and practices. San Diego: Academic; 1993. p. 3–44.
276. Wilcox AJ. Molecular epidemiology: collision of two cultures. Epidemiology. 1995;6(5):561–2.
277. Grandjean P. Biomarkers in epidemiology. Clin Chem. 1995;41(12 Pt 2):1800–3.
278. Ioannidis JP, et al. A network of investigator networks in human genome epidemiology. Am J Epidemiol. 2005;162(4):302–4.
279. Ioannidis JP, et al. A road map for efficient and reliable human genome epidemiology. Nat Genet. 2006;38(1):3–5.
280. Jablonka E. Epigenetic epidemiology. Int J Epidemiol. 2004;33(5):929–35.
281. Manolio TA. Genomewide association studies and assessment of the risk of disease. N Engl J Med. 363(2):166–76.
282. Hunter DJ, Kraft P. Drinking from the fire hose – statistical issues in genomewide association studies. N Engl J Med. 2007;357(5):436–9.
283. Venter JC, et al. The sequence of the human genome. Science. 2001;291(5507):1304–51.
284. McPherson JD, et al. A physical map of the human genome. Nature. 2001;409(6822):934–41.
285. McKusick VA, Ruddle FH. A new discipline, a new name, a new journal. Genomics. 1987;1(1):1–2.

286. McKusick VA. Genomics: structural and functional studies of genomes. Genomics. 1997;45(2):244–9.
287. Hoheisel JD. Microarray technology: beyond transcript profiling and genotype analysis. Nat Rev Genet. 2006;7(3):200–10.
288. Kronick MN. Creation of the whole human genome microarray. Expert Rev Proteomics. 2004;1(1):19–28.
289. Anderson NL, Anderson NG. Proteome and proteomics: new technologies, new concepts, and new words. Electrophoresis. 1998;19(11):1853–61.
290. Schulz-Knappe P, et al. Peptidomics: the comprehensive analysis of peptides in complex biological mixtures. Comb Chem High Throughput Screen. 2001;4(2):207–17.
291. Hegde PS, White IR, Debouck C. Interplay of transcriptomics and proteomics. Curr Opin Biotechnol. 2003;14(6):647–51.
292. Nobeli I, Thornton JM. A bioinformatician's view of the metabolome. BioEssays. 2006;28(5):534–45.
293. Xiong M, et al. A systems biology approach to genetic studies of complex diseases. FEBS Lett. 2005;579(24):5325–32.
294. Ulrich CM, Nijhout HF, Reed MC. Mathematical modeling: epidemiology meets systems biology. Cancer Epidemiol Biomark Prev. 2006;15(5):827–9.
295. Nicholson JK. Global systems biology, personalized medicine and molecular epidemiology. Mol Syst Biol. 2006;2:52.
296. Toscano WA, Oehlke KP. Systems biology: new approaches to old environmental health problems. Int J Environ Res Public Health. 2005;2(1):4–9.
297. Anthony JC. The promise of psychiatric enviromics. Br J Psychiatry Suppl. 2001;40:s8–11.
298. Heyman B. Risk, safety and clinical practice : health care through the lens of risk. Oxford/New York: Oxford University Press; 2010. x, 257 p.
299. Clermont G, et al. In silico design of clinical trials: a method coming of age. Crit Care Med. 2004;32(10):2061–70.
300. Whitcomb DC, et al. Evaluating disorders with a complex genetics basis. The future roles of meta-analysis and systems biology. Dig Dis Sci. 2005;50(12):2195–202.
301. Rothman N, Stewart WF, Schulte PA. Incorporating biomarkers into cancer epidemiology: a matrix of biomarker and study design categories. Cancer Epidemiol Biomark Prev. 1995;4(4):301–11.
302. Boffetta P. Molecular epidemiology. J Intern Med. 2000;248:447–54.
303. Mechanic LE, et al. Next generation analytic tools for large scale genetic epidemiology studies of complex diseases. Genet Epidemiol. 2012;36(1):22–35.
304. Boffetta P, Islami F. The contribution of molecular epidemiology to the identification of human carcinogens: current status and future perspectives. Ann Oncol. 2013;24(4):901–8.
305. Schunemann HJ, et al. Letters, numbers, symbols and words: how to communicate grades of evidence and recommendations. CMAJ. 2003;169(7):677–80.
306. Atkins D, et al. Grading quality of evidence and strength of recommendations. BMJ. 2004;328(7454):1490.
307. Guyatt GH, et al. GRADE guidelines 17: assessing the risk of bias associated with missing participant outcome data in a body of evidence. J Clin Epidemiol. 2017;87:14–22.
308. Schunemann HJ, et al. GRADE guidelines: 16. GRADE evidence to decision frameworks for tests in clinical practice and public health. J Clin Epidemiol. 2016;76:89–98.
309. Andrews JC, et al. GRADE guidelines: 15. Going from evidence to recommendation-determinants of a recommendation's direction and strength. J Clin Epidemiol. 2013;66(7):726–35.
310. Andrews J, et al. GRADE guidelines: 14. Going from evidence to recommendations: the significance and presentation of recommendations. J Clin Epidemiol. 2013;66(7):719–25.
311. Guyatt GH, et al. GRADE guidelines: 13. Preparing summary of findings tables and evidence profiles-continuous outcomes. J Clin Epidemiol. 2013;66(2):173–83.

312. Guyatt GH, Oxman AD, Schunemann HJ. GRADE guidelines-an introduction to the 10th-13th articles in the series. J Clin Epidemiol. 2013;66(2):121–3.
313. Brunetti M, et al. GRADE guidelines: 10. Considering resource use and rating the quality of economic evidence. J Clin Epidemiol. 2013;66(2):140–50.
314. Guyatt GH, et al. GRADE guidelines: 12. Preparing summary of findings tables-binary outcomes. J Clin Epidemiol. 2013;66(2):158–72.
315. Guyatt G, et al. GRADE guidelines: 11. Making an overall rating of confidence in effect estimates for a single outcome and for all outcomes. J Clin Epidemiol. 2013;66(2):151–7.
316. Guyatt GH, et al. GRADE guidelines 6. Rating the quality of evidence – imprecision. J Clin Epidemiol. 2011;64(12):1283–93.
317. Guyatt GH, et al. GRADE guidelines: 7. Rating the quality of evidence – inconsistency. J Clin Epidemiol. 2011;64(12):1294–302.
318. Guyatt GH, et al. GRADE guidelines: 5. Rating the quality of evidence – publication bias. J Clin Epidemiol. 2011;64(12):1277–82.
319. Guyatt GH, et al. GRADE guidelines: 8. Rating the quality of evidence – indirectness. J Clin Epidemiol. 2011;64(12):1303–10.
320. Guyatt GH, et al. GRADE guidelines: 9. Rating up the quality of evidence. J Clin Epidemiol. 2011;64(12):1311–6.
321. Guyatt GH, et al. GRADE guidelines: 4. Rating the quality of evidence – study limitations (risk of bias). J Clin Epidemiol. 2011;64(4):407–15.
322. Balshem H, et al. GRADE guidelines: 3. Rating the quality of evidence. J Clin Epidemiol. 2011;64(4):401–6.
323. Guyatt G, et al. GRADE guidelines: 1. Introduction-GRADE evidence profiles and summary of findings tables. J Clin Epidemiol. 2011;64(4):383–94.
324. Guyatt GH, et al. GRADE guidelines: 2. Framing the question and deciding on important outcomes. J Clin Epidemiol. 2011;64(4):395–400.
325. Pottie K, et al. GRADE equity guidelines 4: guidance on how to assess and address health equity within the evidence to decision process. J Clin Epidemiol. 2017;90:84–91.
326. Akl EA, et al. GRADE equity guidelines 2: considering health equity in GRADE guideline development: equity extension of the guideline development checklist. J Clin Epidemiol. 2017;90:68–75.
327. Welch VA, et al. GRADE equity guidelines 1: health equity in guideline development-introduction and rationale. J Clin Epidemiol. 2017;90:59–67.
328. Welch VA, et al. GRADE equity guidelines 3: health equity considerations in rating the certainty of synthesized evidence. J Clin Epidemiol. 2017;90:76–83.
329. Buhn S, et al. The risk of bias in systematic reviews tool showed fair reliability and good construct validity. J Clin Epidemiol. 2017;91:121–8.
330. Laszlo A, Krippner S. Systems theories: their origins, foundations, and development. In: Jordan JS, editor. Systems theories and a priori aspects of perception, vol. 126: North Holland; 1998. p. 47–74.
331. Diez Roux AV. Complex systems thinking and current impasses in health disparities research. Am J Public Health. 2011;101(9):1627–34.
332. Sterman JD. Learning from evidence in a complex world. Am J Public Health. 2006;96(3):505–14.
333. Bar-Yam Y. Improving the effectiveness of health care and public health: a multiscale complex systems analysis. Am J Public Health. 2006;96(3):459–66.
334. Galea S, Riddle M, Kaplan GA. Causal thinking and complex system approaches in epidemiology. Int J Epidemiol. 2010;39(1):97–106.
335. Hu JX, Thomas CE, Brunak S. Network biology concepts in complex disease comorbidities. Nat Rev Genet. 2016;17(10):615–29.
336. Harding SG. Can theories be refuted?: essays on the Duhem-Quine thesis, Synthese library, vol. 81. Dordrecht-Holland/Boston: D. Reidel Pub. Co.; 1976. xxi, 318 p.
337. Duff A. Pascal's wager and infite utilities. Analysis. 1986;46(2):107–9.
338. Gruer L, Hart CL, Gordon DS, Watt GC. Effect of tobacco smoking being associated with a two to fourfold increased mortality risk, even when adjusted for social position: a 28 year cohort study. BMJ. 2009;338:b480.

Index

O. Dammann, B. Smart, *Causation in Population Health Informatics and Data Science*, https://doi.org/10.1007/978-3-319-96307-5

MIX
Papier aus verantwortungsvollen Quellen
Paper from responsible sources
FSC® C105338

If you have any concerns about our products,
you can contact us on
ProductSafety@springernature.com

In case Publisher is established outside the EU,
the EU authorized representative is:
Springer Nature Customer Service Center GmbH
Europaplatz 3, 69115 Heidelberg, Germany

Printed by Libri Plureos GmbH
in Hamburg, Germany